The Concussion Cure

3 Proven Methods to Heal Your Brain

Paul Henry Wand, MD

The Concussion Cure: 3 Proven Methods to Heal Your Brain

Copyright © 2019 by Paul H. Wand, MD

All rights reserved.

ISBN: 978-1-7331435-0-9 (print)
ISBN: 978-1-7331435-1-6 (ebook)

Printed in the United States of America

Website: www.theconcussioncure.com
Email: paulwandmd@gmail.com
Phone: 954-344-9772

Editing: Jessica Vineyard, Red Letter Editing, www.redletterediting.com.

Preface

By the time we graduate high school most of us had schooling in what the heart was. If not in biology class then through conversation about open heart surgery, or people we knew who had heart attacks, most of which were caused by blood clots, creating ischemia in the heart muscle (lack of oxygen). But whoever heard of a brain attack? "Your Aunt Sophie had a brain attack." Virtually no one. But in 2014, according to the CDC over 2.8 million visits to a hospital emergency departments were due in whole or in part to concussion or traumatic brain injury. And over 800,000 of these were children. Currently as of 2018, the CDC states *we miss approximately 8 of every 9 concussions,* **or 88% go undiagnosed, over 7 million children and 18 million adults.** And the numbers are rising which makes it a threat to public health. So much show that the CDC is putting together a National Surveillance Concussion System. Its fate in the Trump budget is unknown.

We don't talk about brain attacks because concussion is not nearly as dramatic as a heart attack. And it often goes unseen and undetected by physicians and lay people alike. The people who suffer do so mostly in silence and most are unaware of their injury and/or the injury's relation to trouble in their lives. In the nearly 39 years of practice I would say that half the patients who present in my office with complaints and have a QEEG turn out of have, *currently an undiagnosed* post-concussion syndrome that they are unaware of. I would say that our numbers vastly underestimate this health problem, its incidence and severity and longevity. Research shows that it may take 10 years for symptoms to appear! By that time most people may have forgotten about the actual index injury.

When I worked on the mental health unit of the Juvenile Detention Center in Miami, Florida my job was to provide psychological evaluations of juveniles, 12-17, on that unit. Most of the findings were expected, conduct disorder, depression, anxiety, ADHD, learning disorders. But, **the most unexpected finding was that 80%, at least, of the inmates had post-concussion syndrome**. I called the State Attorney's office and spoke to the assistant SA (State attorney or DA in other states) in charge of these children. His response was, "So what?" I said, "Well you could treat them and make it lot less likely that they will re-offend." After all these were mentally ill children diagnosed with objective testing. He said, "That's not my job. My job is to lock them up and keep them there." Shameful. Most of the children received their head injuries at the hands of their parents who were hitting them and fights they got into on the streets of Miami.

Now you understand why this book is so important. Why you must read it and pass it around to family and friends. Discuss it on a date or give your date a copy. Tell your hairdresser, barber, butcher, police officer or the most unexpected people. Education is the key to saving lives and improving the quality of our lives and the lives of those around us.

Dr. Wand has done us all a favor by writing this book. Return the favor by spreading the word.

Gerald Gluck, Ph.D. LMFT, Board Certified Biofeedback-Neuro, (BCN) Senior Fellow-2

Coconut Creek, Florida 33066

Contents

Introduction

Kenney Bui loved playing football for Evergreen High School in the verdant city of Seattle, Washington. When he was six years old, he began watching the Seattle Seahawks with his dad and became a serious fan, so when he made the football team at seventeen years old, he was living his dream.

During a game on September 4, 2015, he suffered a mild concussion and complained of a minor headache. His coach removed him from the game. Thirteen days later he was cleared to play again.

On October 2, almost exactly a month later, Kenney was tackled during another game. This time he left the field right away, complaining of a severe headache. Then he lost consciousness. Kenney never woke up, and he was taken off life support three days later. He died as a result of a traumatic brain injury.

Traumatic brain injuries, or TBIs, can happen any time, anywhere, to anyone. Whether the injury is minor, from falling off a bicycle, or major, from a devastating car accident, brain injuries can lead to long-term problems and even death if not appropriately treated.

As a neurologist, I have treated thousands of brain injuries over more than three decades. During that time, I developed a treatment protocol that has resulted in truly remarkable reversals of the consequences of brain damage and possibly even regenerates brain tissue.

From a young man who dropped out of university when his grades declined as a result of several minor concussions as a child, to a young woman who had been confined to a wheelchair for nine years after a severe car accident, my patients come in with injuries that cover the entire range in severity and age. In every case, their improvements make significant differences in their lives, often dramatically so. After treatment, the man successfully went back to university, and the woman was able to walk up stairs with assistance.

These cases are discussed in detail.

I became fascinated with the brain while in medical school. During that time, my passion for research was ignited, and it has continued to burn brightly throughout my medical career of forty-plus years. I continue to be fascinated with the brain's remarkable ability to heal and regenerate tissue.

After completing my residency in neurology in 1982, I went into private practice in South Florida, and soon applied my skills in basic research to clinical neurology research. In 1987, I learned new methods of performing diagnostic brain scans, called *QEEG* (quantitative electroencephalogram) and *QEP* (quantitative evoked potentials), and in 1990, I learned of a new diagnostic test to image the brain, called *SPECT*. Now I had three different diagnostic tests to prove and document traumatic brain injuries.

I was the only neurologist in my county performing these diagnostic tests, and thus I became a pioneer in the field of TBI. As the years progressed and I continued my research and learning, I added other modalities of treatment to my protocol. Around the same time I learned about SPECT, I began using hyperbaric oxygen therapy (HBOT) and supplements to treat my patients with brain injuries, and in 2007 I added neurofeedback, a treatment modality that corrects any abnormal brain waves by retraining the brain using a reward system.

I decided to write a book on concussion to share the highly effective methods I have used to evaluate, treat, and enable my patients to recover from traumatic brain injury with a wider audience. I have not published my work beforehand because as a private practitioner working full time in an office and in several hospitals to see patients, there is a time constraint on how much I can do, and the resources required to perform clinical trials are typically available in academic settings, which I am not now a part of.

It is very difficult for a physician in private practice to conduct a clinical trial in an office setting, and in fact there is fierce competition with academicians to work with the pharmaceutical companies (assuming a drug trial). I have to admit that I never even had the idea to write this book until I had a sudden epiphany and realized that I must write it, because it would be the only way to get my message out to the general public.

The Concussion Cure offers a wealth of information on how the brain functions, what the mechanisms of injury to the brain are, and how to diagnose and treat concussions, all of which have a major impact on reversing the symptoms of a concussion.

This book is for those who have suffered a brain injury (or many minor injuries), their families and friends, and anyone who is interested in being prepared for the possibility of brain concussion in the future, such as parents of middle and high school sports players, including football players. Patients must take control of their own health education to benefit from the advances in modern medicine and technology, and my goal is to inform you on how to do just that regarding concussion.

When you finish reading this book, you will have gained state-of-the-art knowledge about:

- how to recognize the symptoms of a concussion.

- how to request the most accurate diagnostic tests from your doctor.

- what medication to ask for and what supplements you should take.

- when to request therapeutic neurofeedback.

- how to request hyperbaric oxygen therapy (HBOT).

Part I discusses the definition of a concussion, describes what goes wrong in the brain after a concussion, and explains the anatomy of the brain. Part II describes how any concussion can be diagnosed with advanced diagnostic tools. Part III discusses the powerful healing treatments I have used to treat brain injuries, including prescribing a specific FDA-approved medication, having patients undergo oxygen treatment such as HBOT, and having them use neurofeedback to retrain the brain. I have included several case studies with links to videos showing patients before and after treatment.

If you or a loved one is suffering from the effects of a traumatic brain injury, I encourage you to read the entire book, make notes, and talk to your doctor. Ask your doctor to order the tests I recommend, and then get them done. By doing so, you can take control of your treatments using my protocol, and you will most likely see dramatic improvements in the health of your brain.

Part I: Understanding Concussions

Chapter 1

What Is a Concussion?

Many people have no idea what a concussion actually is. The modern definition of concussion is a head injury that temporarily interrupts brain activity. It can be caused by a blow to the head or by a force applied to the body that transfers to the head. There may be a loss of consciousness, but not always.

Concussions are graded based on the severity of the force applied. In a grade one concussion, there is no loss of consciousness (LOC); in a grade two, there is a LOC of less than thirty minutes; and in a grade three, there is a LOC of greater than thirty minutes, which typically means that the person is in a coma.

There are many ways by which a person may sustain a concussion. Obvious examples include head-to-head crashes, such as those in professional football; direct blows to the face or head, such as boxers receive; blunt weapons or fists to the face or head; falls, such as slip-and-falls; falls from heights, such as falling off a horse; motor vehicle accidents in which the head strikes a window or another part of the vehicle (or even another occupant); and any type of movement that causes acceleration/deceleration forces to the brain. A less common and less obvious cause is whiplash injury, which occurs when the head and neck move rapidly forward and backward, creating an acceleration/deceleration force that is absorbed by the brain.

The brain

The brain is divided into two halves called *hemispheres*. Each hemisphere is subdivided into four sections called *lobes*: frontal, parietal, temporal, and occipital. Each lobe is responsible for a different set of functions. The frontal lobe, at the front of the brain, is in charge of cognitive function and voluntary movement of the body. The parietal lobe, which sits at the crown of the brain, processes information about touch, movement, taste, and temperature, while the temporal lobe processes memories and associates them with the senses of taste, touch, sound, and sight. The occipital lobe, at the back of the brain, is responsible for vision.

The brain floats inside the skull in a substance called *cerebrospinal fluid* (CSF). The CSF acts as a barrier between the bony skull and the delicate, soft, gelatinous substance that makes up the brain. The brain is not fixed inside the skull, and consequently, it is susceptible to the forces of acceleration, deceleration, and twisting movements.

The frontal lobe floats freely within the skull, so this part of the brain moves more than the other parts and thus absorbs a greater impact than the rest of the brain when a force is applied to the head or neck. This is why we see maximal damage in the front of the brain, with a gradually decreasing gradient going back toward the rear parts of the brain.

A brain injury occurs in a gradient, from superficial to deep, based on the severity of the force. Thus, in mild injuries, the front portion and the superficial layers of the brain are always impacted, whereas in severe injuries, the damage occurs or starts in the frontal and temporal lobes and continues inside the brain to the deeper structures, such as the brainstem and the rear parts of the brain.

The brain stem is the structure that functions as a relay station for information going from the brain to the spinal cord and from the body to the brain. In more severe cases, when the brainstem is involved, concussion is typically accompanied by a loss of consciousness, fractured skull, coma, and various types of bleeding.

As the brain moves back and forth, it can also move in a twisting motion. Thus, it can twist in a quasi-circular manner, which causes a shearing effect and resultant injury. The cerebral cortex, also called *grey matter*, sits on the top of the brain. It has a different tissue density than the structures below it. A twisting motion creates a force that is absorbed by the place where these two parts of the brain, the cortex and the structures below, meet. The structure at this interface is called *white matter*. White matter conveys electrical signals from the cortex to the other parts of the brain. A twisting force can damage and tear the delicate fibers of the white matter.

This type of damage is located specifically where the grey matter and the white matter below it meet, and is called a *diffuse axonal injury*, or DAI. This type of injury comes in two varieties: hemorrhagic DAI, which includes bleeding, and non-hemorrhagic DAI, with no bleeding.

Traumatic brain injuries can easily be overlooked when other injuries are present. An example is a concussion that occurs during a motor vehicle accident in which the occupant sustains multiple injuries. Often with these cases, the injured person goes to the emergency room (ER) and complains about the most painful parts of the body, typically the neck, back, or both, so these are the areas that draw the ER doctor's attention. As a result, the brain injury is overlooked. The patient is discharged from the ER and then undergoes a series of treatments, such as physical therapy, to relieve the dominant pain. The brain injury continues to go undetected.

After several months of therapy and with gradual healing of the pain, the patient stops taking pain medications, which often have side effects on cognitive functioning and can mask symptoms of concussion. Once the patient is off the medications, evidence of the brain injury begins to become evident. They may become forgetful, have trouble concentrating, and make mistakes at work.

At this point, six to nine months have passed since the injury, and the patient goes to a physician for an evaluation of the cognitive decline. Since so much time has elapsed since the accident, the patient doesn't relate these symptoms to the collision, so the physician has to be astute and look for a history of trauma. This is why concussions are so often overlooked and go untreated.

As a free-floating organ inside the skull, the brain is susceptible to damage from forces that impact the body and the head itself. Resulting concussions can easily be overlooked by attending physicians, yet this knowledge can help a concussion sufferer guide their own examinations after a forceful impact.

Chapter 2 looks at the various ways that a concussion physically damages the brain.

Chapter 2

How a Concussion Damages the Brain

A head injury can cause many types of damage to the brain. Much of this damage is determined by the structure of the various tissues that make up the brain.

During the injury event, whatever its cause, the brain is jolted around inside the skull and absorbs the forces it is subjected to. These forces cause the brain to strike against the inside surface of the skull, called the *inner table*. As explained in chapter 1, the maximal force applied to the brain is almost always in the front, and so it is the frontal and temporal lobes that bear the brunt of the injury. The back of the brain is usually the least affected, but this area is not immune to damage.

Hypoperfusion and ischemia

Many things happen as a result of the acceleration/ deceleration effect that cause a brain injury. First and foremost, there is a relative narrowing, or spasming, of the arteries, which causes a decrease in blood flow known as *hypoperfusion*. This reduces the oxygen carried by the arteries to the cells of the brain, resulting in a condition known as *ischemia* (not enough oxygen-rich blood). These two terms will be used throughout the discussions on TBIs.

Cells in the brain called *neurons* are very sensitive to oxygen, and as little as a 20 percent reduction of blood flow can result in what is called *neuronal dysfunction*. This is when the ischemic neurons do not function properly, which in turn causes the many symptoms commonly seen in concussions.

A person who has suffered a concussion might have the typical symptoms of headache, dizziness, impaired memory, ringing in the ears (tinnitus), difficulty performing simple math, speaking and comprehending (aphasia), and have difficulty performing higher cognitive functions such abstraction, planning, and executive functions (memory, self-control, and mental flexibility). They may also experience personality changes, irritability, aggressive behavior, depression, anxiety, and left-right confusion, to name the most common symptoms.

The spasming of the arteries, and especially of the smaller-diameter arteries called *arterioles*, is a widespread phenomenon throughout the brain after an injury. This spasming is more severe in the presence of bleeding, which then causes the concussion to be more severe. The arteriolar narrowing most likely occurs even without bleeding (which can be determined by imaging the brain with a CT scan or the more sensitive MRI if there is enough macroscopic bleeding), although it is not possible to image microscopic bleeding with current state-of-the-art equipment.

Bleeding in the brain complicates a concussion. A good example of this is seen in cases with a type of bleeding called *subarachnoid hemorrhage*, which may produce a secondary stroke after the initial injury. Autopsy studies show there is always microscopic damage after a concussion, so it is likely that there is always microscopic bleeding after concussion that goes undetected. The hypoperfusion that is the consequence of arteriole spasming is, in my opinion, the hallmark injury to the brain, but it is often ignored by practitioners who see and treat this kind of patient.

Hypoperfusion and the resulting ischemia immediately cause neuronal dysfunction in the rest of the neurons, as described previously. As a result, the communication between cells and groups of cells called *hubs* becomes impaired. These hubs are specific to individual brain functions and are identified by tests such as functional magnetic resonance imaging (fMRI) and quantitative electroencephalography (QEEG). Communication between cells and hubs may be impaired in different ways, such as an increase or decrease in the speed of communication. (See chapter 7 for more on QEEG and impairments of the brain's electrical function.)

Another type of impairment is of a metabolic nature, which may be best described as a "cascade of events." Neuronal membranes surround the neurons and allow them to produce electrical signals called *potentials*, which travel along the membranes. When the abrupt ischemia from a brain injury affects the neuron, the neuronal membrane suffers damage as well, which in turn damages structures on the membrane called *channels*, including a very important one called the *calcium channel*.

Calcium channels

Channels are the functional and structural microscopic areas on the cell membrane that control the flow of chemicals such as charged particles like sodium, potassium, and calcium. When the calcium channel is damaged, it allows an excessive inflow of calcium, which in turn causes damage inside the cell and eventually cell death.

Cell death results in inflammation, cellular debris, and oxidative stress, all of which promote further damage to the brain's injury. While the brain has mechanisms to clean up this damage, it can become overwhelmed and may require external assistance in the form of anti-inflammatories and other supplements to rebuild the basic neuronal structures, including the membranes.

A concussion damages the brain in a variety of ways, both macroscopically and microscopically. Many types of damage can lead to the death of neurons, which in turn can cause debilitating loss of cognitive and physical functions. The next chapter explores more deeply the tpes of brain damage caused by a concussion.

Chapter 3

Types of Brain Damage
from a Concussion

We have seen how a concussion damages the brain, and many different types of damage occur as a result, depending on the location and severity of the injury. Before we can understand the types of damage to the brain, however, we must have some basic understanding of the brain's normal anatomy.

The brain has two general anatomical parts: gross anatomy and microscopic anatomy. This chapter addressed gross anatomy, which is the parts that can be seen by the naked eye. A discussion on microscopic anatomy and brain damage is found in chapter 6.

The brain sits inside the skull and is surrounded by the cerebrospinal fluid (CSF). The CSF acts as a buffer, or cushion, which lessens traumatic forces by absorbing and dissipating the energy of the blow. However, there is a limit to how much force it can deflect, and when that threshold is exceeded, the brain sustains injury. As mentioned in chapter 2, it moves in many directions and gets pushed and squashed against the inside surface of the skull until the force is completed absorbed.

The brain is also protected by a series of membranes, the most important of which is called the *dura mater*. The dura mater is the most external layer of the brain and sits tightly against the inner table of the skull. The arachnoid is located beneath the dura and extends through a space above the surface of the cortex. The next layer, the pia, is a discrete lining on the surface of the cortex. Since the entire brain is covered in blood vessels that are fragile and vulnerable to any trauma, a force applied to the head is often sufficient enough to rupture the blood vessels, resulting in bleeding on the surface and many other parts of the brain.

The external part of the brain, the part covered by the membranes, is called the *cerebral cortex*. Humans have the largest cortex of all species. Underneath the cortex are the subcortical structures, including the thalamus, a complex relay station that sends signals from the brain to the spinal cord and from the spinal cord to the cerebral cortex. Surrounding the thalamus is the basal ganglia, whose primary function is to control motor movements.

Another part of the brain that, like the membranes, is not composed of brain tissue is called the *ventricular system*. This system consists of open spaces within the various lobes of the brain and contains CSF, which is produced by the pineal gland. CSF is in communication with the subarachnoid space. As mentioned previously, it provides a cushion around the brain and helps to protect the brain from sudden and forceful movements. The subarachnoid space at the bottom of the brain is in communication with the subarachnoid space in the spinal cord.

The brain's structure can be categorized by classifying discreet parts based on the kind of tissue they contain. Thus, the grey matter is primarily found in the cerebral cortex (although there are some grey structures deeper in the brain), which dominates the surface of the brain. The white matter is primarily beneath the cortex, or subcortical. The grey matter mostly contains neurons and their connections, whereas the white matter mostly contains connecting fibers. The names grey matter and white matter come from the general appearance of the brain once it has been preserved with chemicals (see fig. 1 on following page).

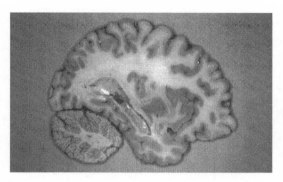

Figure 1

BLEEDING IN THE BRAIN

There are many types of bleeding in the brain, ranging from gross collections of blood called *hematomas* and bleeding into spaces in the brain to microscopic bleeding not visible on routine scanning but verified in autopsy specimens.

Hematomas, always visible to the naked eye, are classified based on their location. The most external and most dangerous type is called the *epidural hematoma*. This injury occurs when an artery between the skull and the dura mater bleeds and creates severe pressure on the brain below. This bleeding is usually rapid since it is coming from an artery, and arteries pump blood strongly in sync with the pumping action of the heart.

As the pressure in the space increases from the expanding mass of blood, it generates a force that pushes downward, literally crushing the soft, gelatinous brain. As the brain is squashed and pushed downward, and because there is no extra space for it to occupy, the cortex and subcortical structures descend lower, eventually squeezing the lowest part of the brain, the brainstem. Once the brainstem is compressed, the patient is comatose and cannot recover. The process of brainstem compression is called *herniation*.

Finally, if the process is not corrected by emergency surgery to relieve the pressure, the victim will remain in a coma and eventually die. The actress Natasha Richardson died of this type of hematoma, which she sustained during a skiing accident at the age of forty-five.

A *subarachnoid hemorrhage* is a type of bleeding named for its location in the subarachnoid space. The blood fills the space, comes in contact with the surface of the brain, and irritates the tissues. In some cases, the blood causes immediate seizures at the scene of the accident.

A type of bleeding called *intraparenchymal hemorrhage* occurs in the substance of the brain. This type of gross bleeding causes considerable damage to the brain because of its mass, compression, increased pressure inside the skull, and irritation due to the blood. The pressure generated by this type of hematoma is potentially dangerous in the same way as the epidural hematoma described previously.

The subdural hematoma (SDH) is so named for its location underneath the dura mater but outside the the arachnoid space below it. Like the epidural hematoma, the subdural hematoma expands and causes pressure on the brain below. The bleeding usually results from a ruptured vein and so bleeding more slowly than the epidural hematoma. Clinically, SDH has three forms: acute, subacute, and chronic.

Acute subdural hematoma

An acute SDH typically appears within hours or days after a blow to the head. The victim is usually aware of the blow and can tell the physician. The patient typically complains of headaches and dizziness, and may report some weakness or clumsiness on the side of the body opposite to where the hematoma is. For example, if the hematoma is in the left hemisphere, the right side of the body could be weak, numb, or uncoordinated.

When the hematoma is in the left frontal lobe, the person may have difficulty speaking, called *Broca's motor aphasia*. If the hematoma is located farther back, in the back of the temporal or the front of the parietal lobe, the person may have difficulty with comprehension, known as Wernicke's or receptive aphasia. The diagnosis is easily made by CT scan or MRI, and the treatment is medical if the hematoma is very small in size but is always surgical if the hematoma is large enough to cause the symptoms just described.

Subacute sudural hematoma

In a subacute SDH, the hematoma starts out very small and does not produce enough compression to cause any symptoms. However, over weeks to perhaps a couple of months, the pool of blood increases, becoming large enough to cause pressure. The same symptoms as described in the acute form then arise. As with acute SDH, when the patient has location-specific symptoms, the treatment has to be surgical evacuation of the blood.

Chronic subdural hematoma

In a chronic SDH, the patient sometimes doesn't know the history of the injury, or the history is vague. The bleeding is slow and progresses slowly over months to a year or so. This is typically the case in older people. An elderly person might strike their head on something and then not recall the injury. This type of hematoma is compounded by the fact that the older population experiences brain atrophy (shrinkage) from aging, which increases the available space that a blood clot can occupy, thereby allowing the hematoma to become larger.

The diagnosis is made when the patient complains of headaches, visual problems, and one-sided weakness. Imaging scans can readily show when the hematoma is on only one side. There are instances when there are hematomas on both sides of the brain, and in this case, diagnosing by using a CT scan may be more difficult because there is no displacement of the brain from one side to the other. An MRI scan of the brain is far superior to CT, and the diagnosis can be easily made. The treatment is always surgical unless there are too many overriding medical problems that would rule out surgery.

Shaken baby syndrome

A particular form of brain trauma worthy of mention, and that is very sad, is called shaken baby syndrome. This injury results when a parent or caretaker holds up a young child, typically an infant, and violently shakes the child back and forth. The baby's head moves back and forth vigorously and rapidly, simulating a whiplash-type injury. Significant trauma and bleeding occur in the baby's underdeveloped brain by the mechanism described previously of how the brain is injured.

Often in these instances, blood enters into the ventricular system, the spaces within the brain that contain CSF. The immaturity of the brain also contributes to the severity of the injury. Other parts of the brain will bleed, as well. The condition often leads to severe, permanent brain damage, including seizure disorder, and is sometimes fatal. A characteristic injury pattern is the diffuse axonal injury, in which the grey matter and the white matter shear.

NEURONS AFTER A CONCUSSION

It is estimated that one neuron in the brain connects with up to ten thousand other neurons, with an estimated total of one trillion synapses in the adult human brain. There are two populations of cells in the brain after a concussion: a group that survives, and a group that eventually dies. The existing connections, or synapses, between the destroyed neurons and the surviving neurons are permanently lost. The neurons that die represent a permanent injury. This is analagous to a stroke, when cells die from lack of oxygen, and a heart attack, when part of the heart dies.

Most importantly, the surviving neurons don't have sufficient blood flow, which then results in ischemia to those cells. These neurons can be treated by increasing oxygen in the cells, which improves metabolic function and can result in a return to normal function, or at least very close to normal. Oxygen treatment is discussed in chapter 10 on hyperbaric oxygen therapy.

POST-TRAUMATIC SEIZURE ACTIVITY

Seizures can happen when a large group of neurons discharges electrical impulses simultaneously and synchronously. Bleeding and red blood cells irritate the cortex and directly contribute to seizure activity, either immediately upon injury or in a delayed fashion.

Seizures are classified into three categories. Immediate seizures are defined as occurring within minutes of an injury. Early post-traumatic seizures occur within the first week and have value in determining a prognosis because their occurrence represents a risk factor for delayed post-traumatic seizures. Late-onset post-traumatic seizures occur more than one week after the injury. Whether a person develops early- or late-type seizures depends on numerous factors such as the severity of the injury, loss of consciousness or length of coma, and bleeding in the brain.

Most seizures emanate from one part of the brain. These are called *focal seizures* and are typical in traumatic brain injuries (TBI), as the injury is frequently worse in specific parts and lobes of the brain. A focal seizure may extend to the rest of the brain in a process called *secondary generalization.*

In a focal seizure, also called a *partial seizure*, the patient never loses consciousness. This type of seizure is not typically associated with motor activity such as involuntary jerking movements of an arm or leg. If the seizure activity emanates from a language area in the dominant hemisphere of the brain, there may be some impairment in the ability to comprehend or speak. Generalized seizures involve both sides of the brain. The patient loses consciousness and may have jerking movements, bite their tongue, and lose control of their bladder or bowels.

I have observed a type of delayed reaction that develops by a process called *kindling*, which can take years to develop and leads to seizure activity. This is a process whereby the damage from the TBI irritates the neurons. They then develop a lowered seizure threshold and thus become more susceptible to an erratic electrical discharge in the brain, which can result in a seizure.

Long-term studies have looked at the delay between the onset of an injury and the development of clinical seizures years later. These longitudinal studies show that the incidence of seizures increases rapidly for the first five years or so after the injury, then plateaus for the next fifteen to twenty years, and then declines for the next five years. This delay of years, coupled with the fact that patients often forget injuries from many years before, makes the diagnosis of post-traumatic seizure disorder easy to miss by the unsuspecting clinician faced with diagnosing the patient.

BRAIN ATROPHY

A normal young brain experiences a natural and progressive loss of neurons called *pruning*. While this process is desirable in the developing brain, it is not desirable in the mature brain. Brain atrophy, or shrinkage of the brain, is a natural process of aging, but a concussion can compound the problem.

As mentioned previously, whenever a single neuron is lost, no matter by what mechanism, it loses contact with ten thousand other neurons. Thus, when a person sustains a concussion and loses that population of neurons, the natural neuronal loss is compounded, which in effect accelerates the overall process of neuron loss. It is this mechanism, perhaps combined with others, that increases the incidence of dementia in patients with post-concussion syndrome (PCS; a set of symptoms that persist after a concussion). Indeed, brain atrophy has been documented by advanced MRI techniques in such patients.

There are many types of injuries to the brain. Most of them involve bleeding, which is always microscopic and in some cases macroscopic, as well. Sometimes urgent care is required, although often people go years before seeking treatment. This delay compounds the difficulty in diagnosing a concussion because the patient may not remember a head injury from the past.

Being aware of the symptoms of a concussion can help the patient inform their physician, who can then properly diagnose and treat a concussion, even if months or years have passed. The next chapter discusses such symptoms.

Chapter 4

Symptoms of a Concussion

A concussion can manifest as many different symptoms, and there are several ways to describe them. This chapter discusses the functions of the brain that are affected.

Since each lobe of the brain is responsible for specific functions, the symptoms that a person with a concussion experiences will depend on which lobe and what part of that lobe is affected. For some functions, the left side and the right side of the lobe each have unique functions. Curiously, no one understands why such specialization, called *lateralization*, exists.

As emphasized in chapter 2 on how the brain is injured, the frontal lobes, and especially the prefrontal lobes, take the brunt of an injury in the majority of cases. Less frequently, in cases with lateral (side) impacts, the temporal lobes may be more affected than the frontal lobes, but both will be impacted.

Lateralization

Lateralization refers to the fact that one lobe or one part of the brain performs a particular function, and no other lobe or part performs that same function. A prime example of lateralization is that of language, which is subdivided into four aspects: expression (speech), comprehension, inflection (tone of voice), and the ability to comprehend inflection.

Speech is typically controlled by the left frontal lobe in a region called the Broca's area, named after Paul Broca, the physician who discovered it. The comprehension of language is controlled in the left hemisphere, in the junction where the back of the temporal lobe meets the front of the parietal lobe. This region is called Wernicke's area, named after Carl Wernicke, the neurologist who discovered it. The ability to raise or lower the melodic pitch of verbal language is controlled by the right frontal lobe. The ability to comprehend the tone of voice is controlled by the rear of the right temporal/front of the parietal lobes. Thus, there are four language areas that all work in concert when they are functioning normally.

THE LOBES OF THE BRAIN

As described in chapter 1, there are four lobes of the brain, and each lobe has a left and right component (see fig. 2). Hence, you will sometimes read "frontal lobes," which refers to both the left and right frontal lobes. Each lobe has a unique function and is impacted in unique ways when an injury is sustained in that region.

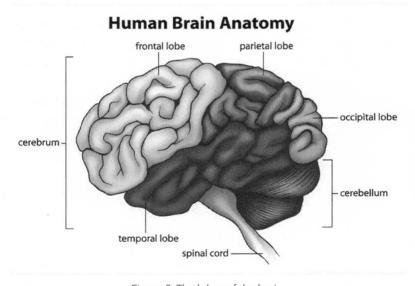

Figure 2. The lobes of the brain.

The frontal lobes

The frontal lobes function in the capacity of what is known as *executive function*. This includes the highest-order thinking, which is observed only in the brains of humans, because we have the most advanced cerebral cortex of all life on Earth. The frontal lobes control abstraction, deduction, advanced planning, motor control, the ability to speak out loud, and emotions.

When the frontal lobe is injured, the person may experience symptoms of depression, suicidal ideation, suicidal attempts, violent behavior, anxiety, memory loss, disorganization, and difficulty in thinking and concentrating. Other symptoms include making errors without realizing it, behaving inappropriately due to the inability to exercise proper judgment, and being ineffectual at completing tasks, which may result in having difficulty maintaining employment or even getting fired.

The temporal lobes

The temporal lobes also demonstrate lateralization, so when the temporal lobe is injured, the person may lose the ability to comprehend speech, to vary the pitch of the voice, and to understand the emotional content of spoken words. An example of the latter is a person who is being yelled at not understanding the person who is yelling at them. The first two impairments are both called *aphasia*.

The parietal lobes

The parietal lobes have some degree of lateralization but not as much as we see in the temporal lobes. Both parietal lobes are involved with the integration of sensory information (visual, tactile, and somatosensory, something that can be felt outside or inside the body, such as warmth) that the brain receives. This information tells us where our body is in space such that we are aware of our surroundings with our eyes closed.

Another function common to both parietal lobes is memory. Some functions are lateralized, such as mathematics, sequencing, and left-right orientation, which are located in the left hemisphere.

Disorders of the parietal lobes include loss of balance, loss of recognition of body parts, difficulty performing math, confusion between left and right, and forgetfulness. When a lesion affects the right parietal lobe, the person may not be aware of the left side of their body, a condition known as *neglect syndrome*.

The occipital lobes

The occipital lobes, located in the back of the brain, are the least affected by concussion. The function of the occipital lobes is primarily related to vision, and visual disturbances are not common in concussion unless there is an injury at that specific location, which can be part of a *coup contrecoup* pattern (an injury that occurs both at the site of trauma and at the opposite side of the brain).

About the only symptom a person could experience in the occipital lobe is a type of loss of vision called *cortical blindness*, in which the person is blind or partly blind and the condition can't be corrected by refractive methods or eye surgery. While it is common for patients to experience other visual symtoms such as double vision, this type of problem comes from other parts of the brain secondary to the trauma.

OTHER SYMPTOMS OF A CONCUSSION

Some classic symptoms of a concussion are almost always present, such as headache, dizziness, nausea, and vomiting but may not be explained by injury to one particular part of the brain. In my decades of experience in practice, I have found that most headaches do not come from the brain but rather from structures such as the neck, cervical spine, and jaw joints.

Occasionally, a patient will report perceiving a headache when they try to think or perform a particular mental function. In this case, the headache may be thought of as coming from the brain, although an argument can be made that when the person is concentrating, they become tense and contract the muscles of the face, which in turn could cause the headache.

Could you have a concussion and not know it?

It is possible to sustain a concussion and never know it, and there are many reasons why this can happen. For example, the person may not develop symptoms until months or years later, and consequently would not make the connection between a remote event and their current symptoms.

Part of the problem can be the person's lack of awareness. If they don't even think they sustained an injury, they won't go to a healthcare provider to be evaluated and can go on to develop symptoms later in life. This is exemplified in case study 4 in chapter 13.

Another example is that the person sustains an injury, goes to the emergency room, undergoes a CT or MRI scan that comes back negative, and then are told they are fine. This is true for about 80 percent of the population, but for the other 20 percent, it is not accurate. If a person did sustain a concussion and the CT or MRI is normal, the scan should be considered a false-negative study, which means that there is indeed a real injury but the test result is considered normal because it is not sensitive enough to detect abnormalities.

Yet another reason one could have a concussion and not know it is when the injured person goes to a healthcare provider with typical complaints of a concussion, a cursory neurological examination does not reveal anything wrong, and the doctor assures the patient that everything is OK. A neurologist may order an MRI scan of the brain (if it is not ordered in the ER), but in the vast majority of mild traumatic brain injury cases (mTBI), the MRI is normal, no injury is diagnosed (false-negative test), and the only treatment recommended is bedrest.

Even less often, the neurologist may order a traditional EEG (electroencephalogram), yet that test will also be normal most of the time.

CONCUSSIONS IN THE NFL

Professional football players in the National Football League (NFL) sustain concussions so often that this topic deserves special attention. Until very recently, a concussion was not considered to be a serious injury. So pervasive was this notion that a player who sustained a concussion was told to just "shake it off" and sent back to play without recovering. Many former players report this exact experience. They also report not recalling what happened in the game after they sustained the concussion.

Concussions have only recently been considered serious injuries that deserve special attention. Despite this, the NFL has been very slow to admit that concussions cause injury and disability to players—especially former players—and even slower to compensate these players, who often become financially insecure despite having earned millions of dollars while playing.

For example, the NFL has instituted a rule that in order for a former player to qualify for a pension, there must be irrefutable evidence of a brain injury as documented by an autopsy. Of all the players who were injured by repetitive blows to the head and body since NFL football has existed, none of them could have satisfied the arbitrary criteria established by the NFL to be eligible to receive benefits.

Dr. Bennet Omalu, a physician, forensic pathologist, and neuropathologist, discovered via autopsies that the brains of several NFL players showed chronic head trauma, which he named *chronic trauma encephalopathy*, or CTE. Using a special technique, he found large accumulations of a substance called *tau protein*, which affects moods, emotions, and executive functions. Unfortunately, the only way to detect the tau protein was during an autopsy.

Several years after Dr. Omalu's discovery, a new type of scan called the *Tau PET* became available. This unique scan can document tau proteins in a living person. Only the Tau PET scan can image a living person's brain in order to show the abnormal accumulation of protein that Dr. Omalu saw microscopically.

To compensate players for their injuries, a lawsuit was settled in 2011 for $765 million. In 2015, a federal judge increased the amount to over one billion dollars. However, there have been issues surrounding the distribution, lawyers are fighting among themselves, and many players or their widows have had their cases disputed by the NFL.

While the NFL serves as a population to study concussions, its players, unfortunately, are paying the ultimate price. However, with the treatment that I recommend, there is hope for current and past players to recover, with the ultimate goal of preventing the development of CTE.

Chapter 5

Concussions in Children

There is a tremendous difference between the brains of children and the mature brains of adults, so pediatric concussions require their own conversation. The pediatric brain is still developing in many ways, including the rapid increase of the number of neurons and the development of a protective coating around nerve fibers called the *myelin sheath*, which is very important for protecting nerve fibers and takes years to completely develop. Another difference is neck strength, which is required to resist the movement of the head and neck in order to dissipate the force applied and reduce the magnitude of a concussion, and which children slowly develop.

Neurosurgeon Robert Cantu wrote a book called *Concussions and Our Kids*, and much of the following information is from this book. Dr. Cantu notes that concussion is a serious matter. For young people age fifteen to twenty-four, sports-related concussion is the second leading cause for concussion behind motor vehicle accidents.

The New York Times reported in 2007 that in the ten years prior to the article, at least fifty young sports players died or were seriously injured from concussion. Dr. Cantu published guidelines about when a player should return to play after a concussion, and many states have adopted such rules, known as "when in doubt, sit them out," for young players.

Dr. Cantu also mentions that ice hockey is more dangerous than previously thought, and methods of concussion prevention include outlawing "checking" to the head in Canada ("checking" describes a defensive technique in hockey). Numerous non-contact sports have been reported to be responsible for concussions, including swimming (being kicked in the head by a fellow swimmer), basketball, volleyball (multiple sub-concussive forces, especially when spiking the ball), wrestling, soccer (where 90 percent of concussions are related to "heading" the ball), baseball (including when a helmet falls off; all helmets are recommended to have chin straps), cheerleading (where the incidence of concussion is ten times greater than for football players), and mixed martial arts.

Dr. Cantu recommends getting a baseline test for players using a test called ImPACT (immediate post-concussion assessment and cognitive testing), which is a simple twenty-minute test for players over the age of twelve. Another test called the King-Devick test examines eye movements and complements the cognitive results of the ImPACT test. Dr. Cantu writes that most concussions resolve in seven to ten days, and most players can return to play in two weeks, but in his practice, about 50 percent of patients do not resolve and instead go on to have post-concussion syndrome. National statistics show that 20 percent of concussions do not resolve.

As discussed previously, Dr. Omalu described the pathology in the brains of NFL players known as chronic trauma encephalopathy. This traumatic consequence of concussion is not limited to adults, and has been identified in young players. A player who died of second-impact syndrome after sustaining a subdural hematoma had autopsy evidence of CTE at the young age of seventeen. One researcher reported that the concussion rate for girls who play high school soccer was 68 percent higher than for boys, and in basketball, boys had concussions at three times the rate for girls.

Dr. Cantu provides the following recommendations to prevent concussions: no tackle football or body-checking in youth hockey before age fourteen, require helmets for field hockey and girls' lacrosse, no heading in soccer until age fourteen, hold sports officials to a higher standard, and require chin straps and restrict head-first sliding for youth baseball. He also recommends that the NFL endorse flag football for youths, which would prevent concussions.

Our children deserve to grow up without suffering preventable head injuries and concussions. By adopting and following these sports guidelines and others particular to specific sports, we will protect our children and do them a great service.

Part II: Diagnosing a Concussion

Chapter 6

The Brain under a Microscope

There are two anatomical parts of brain damage, as mentioned in chapter 3: gross anatomy, injuries that can be seen with the naked eye, and microscopic anatomy, injuries that are visible only through a microscope.

Since the brain is the most complicated organ of the human body, it is no surprise that it has more types of cells than any other organ. There are at least six different cell types in the brain, each of which possess highly specific functions.

For many years, scientists believed that the neurons of the cerebral cortex could not replicate, but that notion has been challenged by modern techniques of analyzing the brain. Now the current thinking is that the brain can produce new cells in specific areas of the brain such as the hippocampus, which is located deep inside the temporal lobe and is thought to be where recent memory is created and stored.

THE CEREBRAL CORTEX

The cerebral cortex, also called grey matter, is the largest portion of the brain and is composed of a varying number of layers, depending on the location. The most advanced type of grey matter is called the *neocortex*, which has six layers. The first layer, near to the surface of the brain, is called the *molecular layer*. It has horizontal connecting fibers, both sensory and motor. The second layer is the *external granular layer* and is predominantly composed of smaller cell bodies. The third layer is the *external pyramidal layer* and is mostly composed of pyramidal cells, and the fourth layer is the *internal granular layer*. The fifth layer is the *internal* (or *ganglionic*) *pyramidal layer*. It contains the largest known pyramidal cells, known as *the cells of Betz*. The last and deepest layer, which is in contact with the white matter below it, is called the *fusiform* or *polymorphic layer*.

The function of the cerebral cortex is quite varied. It is divided into the *sensory cortex*, where the senses of sight, hearing, taste, and smell receive data from the peripheral parts of the body; the *associative cortex*, which sends and coordinates incoming data between lobes (like a central processing unit, or CPU, on a computer); and the *motor cortex*, which contains the fibers that start at the brain, descend to the spinal cord, and go out to the extremities, thus controlling movement.

The variation in the number of layers of cortex accommodate the specialized functions required of each area. As a result, certain areas have a thinner cortex. For example, there are only three layers in the olfactory lobe, which is considered to be a more primitive type of grey matter.

Microscopic regions of the brain

The parts of the lobes that perform various functions are further subdivided into structures known as gyri (singular gyrus). Microscopically, some regions within each gyrus have a characteristic cellular pattern known as cytoarchitecture. These cell patterns were first described by neuroanatomist Korbinian Brodmann, who in 1909 described eighty-eight distinctly different regions (forty-four each on the left and right), with each specific area playing an important role in determining brain dysfunction. Today these regions are known as Brodmann areas.

Brodmann areas play an integral role during neurofeedback treatment to reverse symptoms of a concussion. This very specific and effective type of therapy is discussed in chapter 9.

THE CENTRAL NERVOUS SYSTEM

The central nervous system (CNS) is a complex network of nerve tissues that comprise the brain and spinal cord and that controls the body. There are several different types of signal transmissions in the CNS. For example, in an auditory transmission, when a sound registers in the ear, it is converted to an electrical signal that enters the brain and ends in the part of the brain (the *primary auditory cortex*, or Brodmann area 22) that is responsible for sound. The signal takes only ten milliseconds to go from the ear to the auditory cortex.

In the visual system, the signal starts in the back of the eye, in a structure called the *retina*, and then travels to the back of the brain, where it is interpreted as a visual signal. This process takes about 100 milliseconds and occurs in the *primary visual cortex* (Brodmann area 17). A comparison of the two sensory functions immediately allows one to understand that hearing is ten times faster than seeing.

ABNORMALITIES OF THE CEREBRAL CORTEX

It is a known fact that the brain requires approximately 25 percent of the total blood flow from the heart because of its high metabolic demand, yet it only weighs about two pounds (one kilogram), which is roughly 1 to 2 percent of the total body weight. As you can imagine, there are numerous ways by which the delicate and fragile cortex can be damaged or injured, but here we will address the most common ways.

Stroke is a very common medical condition and is the third leading cause of disability in the United States. Strokes kill about 140,000 Americans each year, which represents one of every twenty deaths annually. Most strokes are of the ischemic type, which means that the artery to that part of the brain becomes blocked, cutting off the blood flow.

Another frequent cause of cortical damage is from trauma from a concussion. Concussions are measured by severity, from the mislabeled mild type, or mTBI, to moderate, and then severe. From an epidemiological and practical point of view, most concussions are classified as the mTBI type. There are millions of cases of mTBI reported each year, and many more that are not reported.

Concussion from sports injuries

There are two general categories of causes of concussion: sports related and non-sports related. In the sports category, more women than men are affected, for example, in soccer, ice hockey, and bobsledding. The opposite is observed in non-sports injuries, where more men are affected.

Most people think of American football as the sport most associated with concussion because of the tremendous forces generated by the athletes, which far exceed the force required for a human to sustain a concussion. Such forces have been studied by Kevin Guskiewicz, the sports director at the University of North Carolina's Sports Medicine Research Laboratory.

In 2008, Guskiewicz's group studied how much force was applied to players' heads and necks by placing small devices called *accelerometers* inside their helmets to measure the forces. Their research showed that concussions occurred at varying degrees of force. They found that some of the low-force impacts caused a concussion, whereas not all of the high-force impacts did.

The g-force a person experiences in a roller coaster or a jet fighter plane is about 4.5g; in a motor vehicle accident at twenty miles per hour, a crash-test dummy hits the windshield at 100g. In football, most of the impacts generate between 20 and 25g, but impacts with forces between 50 and 120g are common, and some are as high as 200g. Guskiewicz's researchers concluded that of the group of sixty football players studied, seven concussions resulted from hits between 100 and 169g, and six resulted from hits less than 85g. These latter findings are in stark contrast to an NFL study that concluded that a force greater than 85g was required to produce a concussion.

In 2002, star NFL player Mike Webster, known as "Iron Mike," died in Philadelphia. He had played for the Pittsburgh Steelers for many years, was a Hall of Famer many times over, and possessed four Superbowl rings. However, Mike suffered from a then-unrecognized brain condition that affected his function and behavior. His brain was severely injured as a result of multiple concussions, which in turn caused him to become depressed, anxious, aggressive, and despondent. He died at the young age of fifty, and an autopsy disclosed that the cause of death was a heart attack.

The neuropathologist who performed the autopsy was Dr. Bennet Omalu, who examined Mike's brain in detail. (This story is depicted in the 2015 movie *Concussion*, starring Will Smith as Dr. Omalu.) When Dr. Omalu viewed slices of Mike's brain tissue under a regular light microscope, he observed peculiarities that had been observed in the brains of boxers but had never before been seen in a football player's brain. The medical term used to describe such a condition in boxers is *dementia pugilistica*, commonly known as punch-drunk syndrome.

The microscopic findings that Dr. Omalu observed, which he coined *chronic traumatic encephalopathy* (CTE), had only been seen in boxers' brains and the brains of older people diagnosed with Alzheimer's disease. In addition to the tau protein deposits and amyloid plaques (clumps of proteins that are the hallmark finding of Alzheimer's disease) in the frontal, temporal, and parietal neocortices (the newest parts of the cortex), he also saw evidence of a loss of neurons in an area of the brainstem called the *substantia nigra*, which is associated with symptoms of Parkinson's disease.

In 2006, Dr. Omalu published a second case of a former NFL player whose brain revealed findings similar to Mike Webster's but did not contain any amyloid plaques. He recommended further study to determine the significance of the findings of CTE in the hope of determining some form of protection and treatment.

Dr. Omalu published a third case in 2010 and again recommended that further long-term studies be done to confirm the common symptoms of CTE in professional American football players.

White matter

Another microscopic finding of importance is in the white matter, the fibers that connect the brain's cells. White matter conducts the electrical signals between the cells and thus provides for their communication. Long-distance communication is vital to the brain's functions, and the connecting fibers in white matter are found between cells at great distances as well as those that are close to each other.

Some of the connections between cells consist of many fibers, which can be seen with the naked eye. These large connections, called *commissures*, extend from front to back and from left to right. The speed of conduction is dependent on the myelin sheath, the protective sheath around the nerve fibers. In general, the thicker the myelin sheath, the faster the signal goes.

Before the current scanning technology was developed, it was impossible to see the microscopic damage done by brain concussions in living people. Fortunately, we can now detect much of this damage with MRI scans, and detect functional abnormalities by QEEG and SPECT scans, which allow for proper detection and treatment of brain injuries.

It is important to know the difference between an EEG test; its derivative, QEEG; and QEP, as well as becoming familiar with the SPECT scan. Many physicians erroneously overlook the latter choices, but these scans are crucial to detecting mild brain trauma in order to treat such injuries properly. The next chapter discusses these vital diagnostic tools so that you or your loved one with a brain injury can be informed and prepared for a discussion with your physician.

Chapter 7

Tools to Diagnose a Concussion

In this chapter, we will look at three important ways to diagnose a concussion: the SPECT scan, the QEEG test, and the QEP test. It is important to know which procedures are recommended to diagnose a concussion and how much experience the physician or test analyzer has in interpreting the data to determine whether or not a concussion has indeed been sustained.

I believe it is crucial for the patient and loved ones to understand how a TBI is diagnosed. The following information is highly valuable to those who have suffered a brain injury, and you are encouraged to learn the difference between the various tests. Once you understand how they are used to diagnose a brain injury, you will be better equipped to request that your physician order them.

Many types of scans can be performed to evaluate an injury to the brain. However, some scans do not offer any meaningful data, while others offer great detail that would otherwise be overlooked.

Scans are informally classified into two categories: those that provide structural information (the physical aspects of the brain), and those that provide functional data (how well a part of the brain is functioning). In the former category are CT and MRI scans. In the latter category is a functional scan called a SPECT scan (*single-photon emission computed tomography*).

STRUCTURAL SCANS

The CT scan became available around 1972, when I was in medical school, and Sir Godfrey Hounsfied is credited with its invention. I recall going to neuroradiology meetings to learn how to read CT scans in 1978, only six years after the scan was developed. The new

CT scan revolutionized brain imaging, since it was the first time the brain of a living person could be seen.

The technology advanced rapidly over the next ten years, during which time CT scanners became more powerful and much more accurate, giving us greater precision in diagnosing any neurological condition that affected the structure of the brain. It also did away with antiquated and uncomfortable imaging methods.

CT scans did much to advance our knowledge of the anatomy of the brain, but they have one particular drawback. Typically, because of how CT scans work, an artifact on the scan is visible where the skull's inner table meets the surface of the brain. As a result, the scan cannot clearly separate the boundary between the two regions. This limitation in CT technology is most often seen where the brain substance is small compared to the bone, such as at the base of the brain, and the brainstem in particular.

Advances in technology are inevitable, and an even more powerful imaging technique known as MRI became available in the late 1970s. It was initially called *nuclear magnetic resonance*, or NMR, because of how it produces images. However, since the word *nuclear* scared people, its name was changed to *magnetic resonance imaging*, or MRI.

I recall when the MRI first became available in my medical community in 1984, only two years after I entered private practice, and how much it improved my ability to make diagnoses. Before this technology, many diagnoses required sometimes painful invasive procedures that were performed only in the hospital.

Over the years, numerous advances and variations in the technology were developed by scientists all over the world, and the MRI and its variants became the main imaging choice over CT scans. The artifact at the interface between bone and brain was no longer there, blood flow in the arteries could be imaged without resorting to dangerous and painful injections of contrast media, and cerebrospinal fluid studies were obtained without performing spinal taps. More advanced methods continued to be invented.

FUNCTIONAL SCANS

The class of functional scans is divided into two subtypes. One is an electrical test of the brain, called *electroencephalography*, or EEG, and the other is the blood flow test, which is the SPECT scan. A discussion on SPECT scans and their value in TBI diagnosis follows.

Invented by nuclear medicine scientist David Kuhl in 1962, the technology for functional scans was originally known as *emission reconstruction tomography*. This same technology formed the basis for both SPECT and PET scans. In 1972, Dr. Kuhl performed the first numerical measurement of blood flow in a human subject. Many variations were developed over the years, and the technology was perfected for different organs of the body.

All of these types of scans require intravenously injecting radio-isotopes into patients before the scan. A radioisotope is an unstable and radioactive form of an element such as iodine or fluorine. These injections have to be approved in the United States by the Food and Drug Administration (FDA). It was not until 1988 that the FDA approved an isotope to perform a brain scan for stroke, which resulted in the SPECT technique lagging far behind the evolution of both CT and MRI.

During those developing years, another nuclear test called *positron emission tomography* (PET) came into use. This test uses some of the same principles as a SPECT scan, although it requires more energy and double the radioactivity. The main advantages of the PET scan are that it measures the metabolic activity of what is injected (typically glucose) and has a higher resolution than the SPECT scan does. However, when it is used to test for mTBI, a PET scan usually returns a normal result, so it is not a useful tool for diagnosing a concussion.

THE SPECT SCAN

I was introduced to the SPECT technology in 1990, and immediately realized that it was a far more sensitive diagnostic test for traumatic brain injuries than CT, MRI, and PET scans. Even when I used the most basic first-generation SPECT scan, which has only one camera head (compared to the modern three-camera scanner), I saw abnormalities that are not visible in the other types of scans. I also noticed that the SPECT scan showed a characteristic pattern for TBI of reduced blood flow (hypoperfusion) in the familiar gradient, with the greatest hypoperfusion in the front parts of the brain and less toward the rear.

After I realized that virtually all of the SPECT scans showed this pattern of hypoperfusion, I postulated that the hypoperfusion could be treated by increasing the blood to the brain. It seems obvious to me now, but back then it was revolutionary and led to a major change in how I treated concussion patients.

The history of the SPECT scan

A brief history of SPECT scans is in order to understand how the current scans were developed, the limitations of the original scanner, and the advancement of the most modern scanners used today to obtain state-of-the-art results.

If a patient wants to have a SPECT scan for their own evaluation, they should be knowledgable about what is available in their local area and make an informed decision to obtain a scan locally, or determine if they have to travel to another city where state-of-the-art scanners are located.

The original scanner has one head, called a camera. The test is performed by injecting a patient with an intravenous radioisotope. The camera then moves around the patient's head as it scans. The single-head camera provides the lowest resolution images compared to more advanced scanners, but it is still a more sensitive test than an MRI. The single-head camera is slower, however; it takes about forty-five minutes to an hour to complete one scan.

Two-camera scanners were eventually developed and cut the scan time almost in half. We now have triple-head cameras, which are even faster and collect more data. As the scanner collects data, the software creates images of slices of the brain into successive planes. The triple-head instruments have much greater resolution, so they are far more precise than the single-head scanner.

HOW A SPECT IS PERFORMED

The patient who is to receive a SPECT scan sits in a dark, quiet room with very little light stimulation, which could cause increased activity in the occipital lobes and lead to a false reading.

The patient is injected intravenously (similar to drawing a routine blood test) with a radioisotope called Ceretec. The amount of isotope used is determined by the patient's weight, and the dose is measured in small amounts called *millicuries* (named after the French scientist Marie Curie, who, together with her husband, Pierre, discovered radioactivity in 1903, for which they were awarded a Nobel Prize). The isotope is "labeled," which means that it emits gamma rays that are then detected by the scanner.

After the injection, the patient is left alone for about thirty minutes to allow for a process called *equilibration*, during which the isotope distributes evenly throughout the brain. The patient then lies on a table for the scan.

Once the scan starts, the cameras rotate around the head, acting like geiger counters to detect the labeled gamma rays after they pass from the inside of the brain to the outside and then exit the skull.

With a single-head instrument, the camera has to move 360 degrees, all the way around the head, to capture all of the gamma rays after they exit the brain and pass through the skull. This is a slow and tedious process, but it is necessary to produce images from all parts of the brain. It also explains why the single-camera scan takes the longest to complete. With the triple-head scanner, each camera moves just 120 degrees, and they all move at the same time, thereby reducing the scan time by a third.

THE SPECT IMAGE

After the scan is complete, the scanner's computer translates the collected data into 2-D and 3-D images of the brain (see figure 3). This has greatly improved our ability to evaluate mTBI because we can now see images of the entire surface of the brain, including the front parts of the frontal and temporal lobes, which are usually the sites of greatest injury in all TBIs.

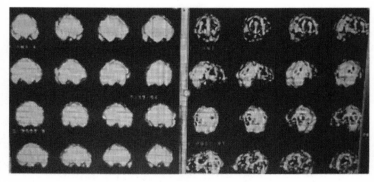

Figure 3. A normal 3-D SPECT scan (left), and a TBI SPECT scan (right)

SPECT 3-D images show in detail the area where the brain received the initial impact of the trauma as it began to shake, twist, and bounce inside the skull. This is a critical area to image and thus far can only be done using SPECT technology.

I used a SPECT scan to image the brain of a patient who had part of a ceiling fall on the left side of his head. Knowing the circumstance of the injury and examining scan images that showed the maximal areas of hypoperfusion, I concluded that the injury was a classic case of a type called *coup contrecoup*, in which the injury causes trauma to both sides of the brain. In this case the brain was shifted by the force applied from the left to the right. As a result, injury was sustained to both the left side and the corresponding right side. The history of the injury event corroborated what I found from the patient's testing, which was helpful in the patient's lawsuit.

If you or someone you know would like to have a SPECT scan done to determine the extent of an injury, it is a good idea to ask for a specific type of scan. Figure 4 shows an example of a prescription you can ask your doctor to write so you can get the scan done correctly.

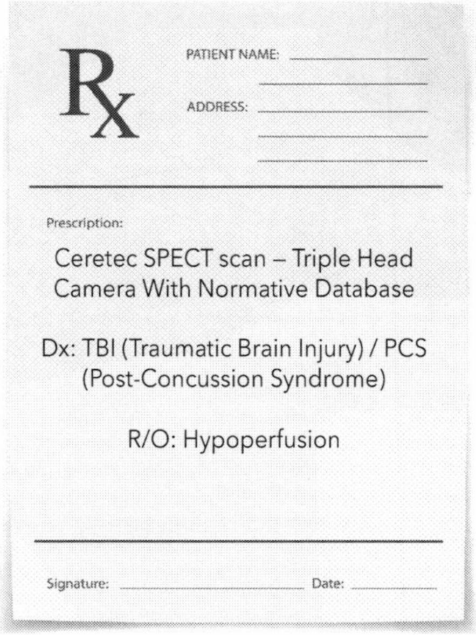

Rx

PATIENT NAME:

ADDRESS:

Prescription:

Ceretec SPECT scan – Triple Head Camera With Normative Database

Dx: TBI (Traumatic Brain Injury) / PCS (Post-Concussion Syndrome)

R/O: Hypoperfusion

Signature: Date:

Figure 4. Sample of a prescription for a SPECT scan.

QEEG

Quantitative electroencephalography, or QEEG, is a computerized quantitative analysis of ongoing brain waves and is another way of looking at the brain for evidence of a TBI. The "quantified" aspect of the data comes from a computerized analysis of the EEG's raw data.

A brief discussion of EEG will help to understand the use of QEEG for diagnosing a TBI.

The EEG

The history of EEG, or electroencephalography, began with the first recording of a human EEG by Hans Berger in 1924. An EEG is done by placing wires called electrodes on the scalp in specific locations, as determined by a method called the *10–20 system*. The numbers refer to the distance between the placement of the electrodes (in percent of the skull's size) after measuring on the scalp.

The scalp is carefully cleaned to ensure a proper connection, and the electrodes are affixed to the scalp. (The hair does not need to be shaved off.) The electrodes are attached to an instrument to amplify the signal and then display the results. Typically, nineteen or twenty electrodes are placed on the scalp. After proper placement and assurance that the contacts with the scalp are good, the electrodes are grouped into specific patterns called *montages*. Different montages are typically arranged and viewed successively.

Performing an EEG

The standard EEG is performed first with the eyes open for at least ten minutes, then with the eyes closed for another ten minutes. One or two "activating techniques" are then performed, such as the patient hyperventilating for three minutes, and finally, a photic stimulation (such as flashing lights) is performed. The purpose of the activating techniques is to elicit an abnormal response even if the rest of the EEG reads as normal.

After the data is collected, it is displayed on a computer screen. An EEG has the appearance of several waveforms and frequencies (see fig. 5). An EEG can be thought of as analogous to the EKG done for the heart but more complicated and with more lines of data.

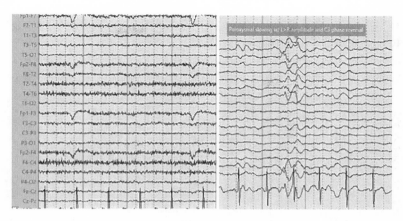

Figure 5a, A normal adult EEG, and Figure 5b, an abnormal EEG (both from my own practice)

The usefulness of EEG data

A raw EEG is traditionally read by visually inspecting it. The interpretation of the raw EEG should be performed only by a physician, typically a neurologist, who is specifically trained to do so, although other professionals may acquire this technical skill.

A routine EEG is helpful in evaluating neurological symptoms, since it provides objective data for a variety of subjective symptoms. It can provide specific and characteristic waveform patterns, which, together with symptoms, can assist in establishing a specific diagnosis. An EEG may also be helpful in monitoring a patient's response to therapy, such as when anti-epileptic medications are prescribed to treat a seizure disorder.

The usefulness of EEG in diagnosing mTBI is limited because most of the results are typically read as normal, thus overlooking possible injury. As a general rule, the more severe a concussion, the greater the probability that the raw EEG will be abnormal. However, there is a caveat to this rule of thumb, which I learned firsthand in 1987 when I began to read and interpret QEEGs.

I observed that most of the patients whom I had diagnosed as having mTBI had an abnormal QEEG, but the raw EEG was normal. When I re-reviewed parts of the raw EEG that was used to create the QEEG, I noted some very subtle changes in the appearance of the brainwaves, known as the background, and often in only one part or side of the brain. I was trained in residency only five years before I began to read QEEG and was taught to consider these subtle findings as normal variants. At the time, we did not have the benefit of QEEG with a *normative database* (a database of many QEEG results that establishes the range of normal—in this case, brains that are free of neuropsychiatric disease).

The lesson I learned was that the subtle changes in the background rhythm were in fact abnormal when analyzed by an objective and scientific normative database. I have since changed my method of reading routine EEGs, and as a result, I find more abnormal EEGs than I used to.

QEEG TECHNOLOGY

Quantitative electroencephalography technology, or QEEG (and sometimes simply Q), became commercially available after advances were made in computer technology, and several models of QEEG instruments burst into clinical practice in the mid-1980s. Prior to that time, QEEG tests were performed but were only available in university centers and only to academicians.

I acquired my first instrument in 1987. It had vast capabilities compared to all prior diagnostic procedures. It could perform QEEG and a full battery of QEP (discussed in the next section). My instrument came equipped with an early-generation 286 CPU. It had a hard drive with a memory of only 40 MB and a large-capacity optical disk to store data. The printer produced color images that took three minutes per page to print, and each study had some twenty to thirty pages. For indefinite data storage, we used disks that had only 10 MB of memory capacity. Over time, I saved many boxes of those disks.

The QEEG procedure

The QEEG test comes from the standard EEG, and thus it starts out like a regular EEG. The "Q" part of the procedure, and what makes this procedure superior to EEG in my opinion, is the fact that QEEG applies a sophisticated analysis to the data, creating a detailed map of the brain. This data is then compared to normative databases that include gender and age. Doing so produces a statistical analysis that objectively shows how abnormal the study is.

For a QEEG procedure, the patient sits in a comfortable chair or lies on their back (mostly when performed in a hospital). As with the EEG, about twenty wires are placed in specific locations on the scalp according to the international 10–20 placement system (see fig. 6). Sometimes a cap with pre-set markers is used in lieu of measuring and marking the locations.

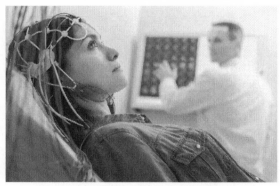

Figure 6. A patient ready for QEEG.

Several types of recordings are made with the patient in various conditions, such as with the eyes open and staring at one spot straight ahead for at least ten minutes, and then with the eyes closed for at least ten minutes. Activating techniques may be performed just as with the EEG.

As with the EEG, various activating techniques can be done, such as hyperventilation and photic stimulation, which are designed to elicit an abnormality, if one exists, by stressing the brain. Hyperventilation, if not medically contraindicated, is carried out for three minutes as tolerated, and then a three-minute post-hyperventilation period is recorded. All of the collected data is stored on a computer.

The technician then visually inspects the tracing, carefully selecting portions that are free of artifacts. Artifacts are waveforms in the tracing that do not come from the brain but rather from sources outside of the brain. These are known as *extracerebral* sources and include eye movements, eye blinks, muscle contractions around the face, heartbeat, and bodily movements, to name the most common.

These artifact-free segments of the raw EEG, which should total at least one minute of data (two to five minutes is preferred), are saved and then subjected to a process called a fast Fourier transformation, or FFT. (The FFT is named after its discover, Baron Jean-Baptiste Joseph Fourier, a mathematician who developed a theory to study the transmission of heat through solids in 1822.)

This entire analysis is performed with the electrodes connected in various patterns. A series of FFT maps, known as voltage maps, are created and stored in the computer. Typically, the maps are in color to show fine details of the electrical changes.

The data then undergoes a statistical analysis. As mentioned previously, the normative database for QEEG consists of normal individuals who are free from known neuropsychiatric diseases and brain dysfunctions. Normative databases are widely used in clinical medicine, and are typically used to establish the limits of "normality" based on a normalized population. They are used in many instances in medical testing such as blood tests, complete blood counts, kidney function, liver function, and many other diagnostic procedures.

For a QEEG test, age is an important factor to consider because of the rapid growth and maturation of the brain in childhood. A

QEEG technician should never attempt to compare data from a senior citizen to a child's data, for example, because the normal brain functions are very different between the two, and a valid comparison cannot be made.

There are many more categories of age in a QEEG normative database than there are in a SPECT normative database, and if the age of the patient getting tested falls outside of the normative range, their data should not subjected to a QEEG analysis. Fortunately, the database I use on my patients has a broad age span, starting from two months after birth to eighty-three years, and is registered with the FDA.

When I started performing and reading QEEGs in 1987, the only parameter to analyze was the FFT, as described. However, over the years, QEEG science and technology have progressed, and other parameters have been added to provide additional informative data on brain function.

LORETA analysis

There are now several complicated quantitative methods of analyzing QEEG, including the powerful LORETA (low-resolution electromagnetic tomographic analysis) method, created by Roberto D. Pascual-Marqui in 1999 and commonly used in QEEG reports. This technique displays the QEEG data in slices, just like MRI scans. Essentially, the LORETA technique employs sophisticated mathematics to determine the origin of events recorded on the surface of the brain but that emanate from sources deep inside the brain.

Knowing whether a localized abnormal electrical discharge that is recorded on the surface of the brain is actually coming from the surface or from deep within the brain is important in diagnosing and treating a condition or mTBI. Thus, the test obtains an image of a slice of the brain just as with MRI except that QEEG examines the electrical data and then compares it to the normative database to establish normal from abnormal. If the data is abnormal, it can be determined how abnormal it is by comparing how far away the data is from the normative database.

As with SPECT, QEEG can show 3-D models of the brain, focusing in on specific areas of the abnormal data from several different views, including the front, the back, the sides, and the mid-line.

PATIENT CASE STUDY: SEIZURE

The case study of patient Judy M. illustrates the diagnostic power of QEEG and demonstrates a program I use to determine the severity of an injury and whether the patient has sustained a TBI.

Judy came in with an existing diagnosis of epilepsy. She told me she had had her first seizure at the age of five, which did not include a fever. (Seizures with fever are common in young children and are related to the fever.) She was hospitalized and evaluated at the time, but no cause for the seizure was found.

Later in her life, Judy started having seizures on a regular basis, and she was treated with the usual anti-epileptic medications. Some of her seizures started with auras (a warning sign that a seizure is coming). They were focal in nature, specifically affecting her right arm. Her neurological examination suggested that there were signs coming from the left frontal lobe of her brain that were consistent with the localization of her auras and her inability to speak during the seizures.

When I saw Judy during her initial consultation, I observed her have a seizure. I noted that she began to have a glazed look in her eyes. Several seconds later, her right shoulder began to twitch, and she started tilting her head to the right. This lasted between thirty and forty seconds, after which she returned back to normal. She did not or could not speak during the episode.

I noted that Judy's medical history was not remarkable, but she did state that she had had a minor head injury during cheerleading, when another girl knocked her down. When she fell, she struck the back of her head on the ground.

Judy had no symptoms to suggest a concussion. My plan of treatment was to obtain a QEEG and SPECT scan. Needless to say, the tests showed objective evidence of a prior TBI, although such testing cannot date the injury. The results of both the SPECT scan and the QEEG tests showed the underlying reason for Judy's seizures.

Her SPECT scan was significantly abnormal. I noted that the study was abnormal because her entire brain showed patterns of hypoperfusion. The hypoperfusion was worse on the left side of her brain than on the right and was specifically in the left central lobe and the right parietal lobe. My overall impression was that the study of Judy's brain was moderately abnormal, with a trauma pattern of coup contrecoup. (see fig. 7).

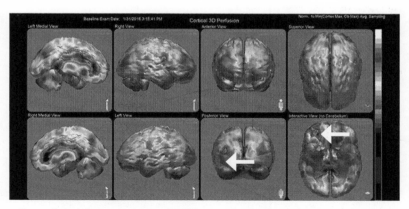

Figure 7. Judy's pre-treatment SPECT scan. The darker areas show severe decrease of perfusion especially in the bottom of the right frontal lobe, and in the back especially in the left greater than right occipital lobes.

The decreased blood flow I observed was statistically significant in the areas described, as well as in the left frontal lobe, where the production of language is located. These findings correlated with other diagnostics I performed with her, such as neuropsychological testing (see fig. 8).

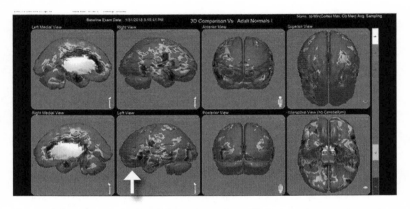

Figure 8. A comparison of Judy's results to that of her normal peers shows that all of thedarker areas show that Judy's blood is less than her normal peers. The arrow points to the language area in her brain that was affected during a seizure, when she could not talk.

We then ran a QEEG test, and I noted that the results were abnormal compared to a normal group of peers, and were especially worse in the left than the right frontal, temporal, and occipital lobes. The results were also abnormal in the parietal lobes, with the right side worse than the left. In general, the QEEG findings corresponded to the SPECT findings.

A powerful technique that is available only in QEEG technology is a mild traumatic brain injury discriminant score, which is an analysis to see if the patient's EEG matches the EEGs of others who have an mTBI. If there is a match with an EEG in the existing databank, the patient is considered to have sustained a TBI. The result is expressed as a percentage, and Judy's discriminant showed a 90 percent probability that she had a TBI.

Another parameter used to evaluate patients is called the traumatic brain injury severity index. The index has both a quantitative (numerical) rating and qualitative rating. Judy's quantitative score was 2.81, and her qualitative score showed a mild injury.A test called the concussion index uses QEEG parameters to assess more severe concussions and to determine changes of concussion over time (see fig. 9). Judy's index placed her in the moderate TBI category.

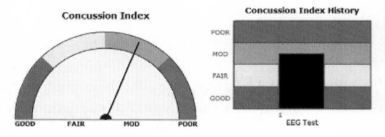

Figure 9. The concussion index.

On the basis of Judy's history and the SPECT and QEEG findings, her diagnosis was a type of seizure that started in one part of her brain and then spread to the rest of the brain. Her diagnosis was therefore changed from epilepsy to what neurologists call *focal seizure disorder with secondary generalization*, quite different from the initial diagnosis of epilepsy. She had one follow-up treatment, at which time I adjusted her medication to better control her ongoing seizures and referred her to neurofeedback.

ADVANTAGES OF QEEG OVER STANDARD EEG

It is clear that the QEEG procedure is far superior to the standard EEG for many reasons, including the following:

1. QEEG is a valid, scientifically accepted diagnostic procedure, documented by hundreds if not thousands of peer-reviewed articles.

2. QEEG is a more sensitive diagnostic than EEG by an estimated 17 percent.

3. The interpretation of QEEG in conjunction with a normative database is a more objective test than a visually interpreted EEG.

4. QEEG permits the analysis of the connectivity between the electrode sites, both locally and at long distance.

5. QEEG permits the true source localization of surface recordings to be determined by a mathematical process called LORETA. Slices in all three planes can be compared directly to MRI and SPECT scans to determine the location of the source. It also permits 3-D imaging, similar to SPECT, which can also be used to determine the actual location of the injury.

6. QEEG helps to formulate a therapeutic program, such as neurofeedback, to be used to retrain the brain due to brain plasticity, or ability of the brain to change.

QEEG is drastically underutilized by neurologists and neurosurgeons for a variety of reasons. To learn more about why this is, see appendix A.

If you or someone you know would like to request a QEEG, you can ask the doctor to write a prescription using the example in figure 10 so the QEEG can be done correctly.

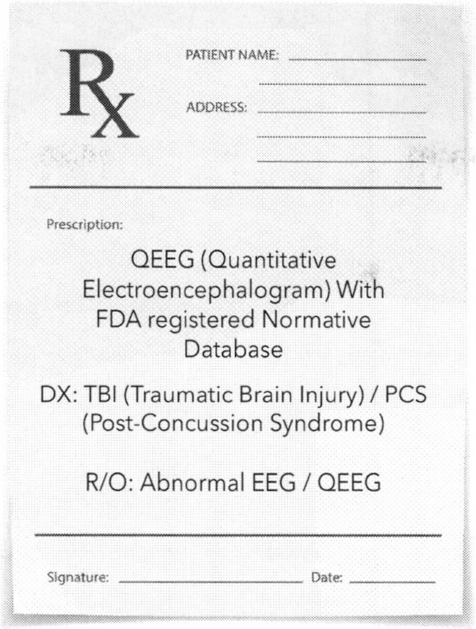

Rx

PATIENT NAME:

ADDRESS:

Prescription:

QEEG (Quantitative Electroencephalogram) With FDA registered Normative Database

DX: TBI (Traumatic Brain Injury) / PCS (Post-Concussion Syndrome)

R/O: Abnormal EEG / QEEG

Signature: Date:

Figure 10. Sample prescription for a QEEG.

THE QUANTITATIVE EVOKED POTENTIAL (QEP)

An evoked potential (EP) is a diagnostic test used to determine if a person has damage to the nerves or the brain. The test has been around since doctors began performing diagnostic testing in the 1950s. The general principle of EP is to stimulate a specific nerve or the brain and record the response. The information appears on a computer screen, numbers are generated, and a doctor reads the results.

The quantitative EP (QEP) test was developed some years later, after computer technology was applied to medical diagnostic testing. When the EP test changed from recording from a single sensor or electrode to employing a full scalp of electrodes, the analysis could be done on specific parts of the brain. In fact, the electrical signal could be traced from the point of stimulation (for example, the eyes or ears) to the primary point in the cortex where the response occurred, and from there followed to other parts of the brain.

There are significant differences between the original EP studies and the subsequently developed QEP studies. The original EPs assess very specific functions, such as vision, sensation, and hearing/balance, and use wires placed on specific parts of the head, arms, or legs. The part of the body on which the wires are placed is specific to the bodily function that is being tested. The response is measured by a computer and interpreted by a physician.

The QEP differs from the EP in that the QEP is performed with a full scalp of wires, whereas the traditional EP uses as few as three, and just one wire in the case of the P300 test. The QEP uses various stimuli, depending on which test is performed. For example, a simple visual evoked potential (VEP), which detects damage to vision nerves or the part of the brain responsible for visual interpretation, is performed with only three wires on the back of the scalp, where the maximal response occurs.

The QVEP

Both the QEP and the QVEP (quantitative visual evoked potential) are performed with nineteen or twenty wires on the scalp, and the response is recorded. Whereas the simpler VEP assesses the visual response just before, at the peak of, and just after the greatest response, the QVEP assesses the same but can also assess the brain's activity after the main response and again after the information goes to other parts of the brain. As we will see in patient Tom B.'s case study (see Chapter 13), the QEP detected an abnormality in the right front part of his brain that would have been completely missed using the routine test.

The QBAER

Another type of EP is an auditory test called *brainstem auditory evoked response* (BAER), which is performed to assess a patient for dizziness. The routine test (without the Q) is performed by placing three wires on the scalp and then positioning headphones over the patient's ears. A series of clicking sounds are delivered to each ear, and each ear's response is recorded by the two channels. The response times are noted and compared to a normative database to see whether the responses are normal or not.

The QBAER is performed with a full scalp of wires, just like the QVEP, and sounds are delivered to each ear through headphones, just like the routine BAER test. The same responses are recorded as in the routine BAER, but in the QBAER, the last response that comes from the cortex is also noted, and that response's activity over the entire scalp is noted.

If there is a delay in the response time, and/or if the amplitude of the response at any of the nineteen wires is 50 percent lower than those of the normative database or a left-to-right comparison, then the test is noted as abnormal. In Tom B.'s case, we will see that the last wave, which the QBAER records but the BAER does not, showed significant asymmetry and helped me make the proper diagnosis.

The P300

The last EP is a cognitive test and is more complicated than the previously described tests. In the P300 routine test, only one wire is used, placed on the top of head. The stimulus can be visual, auditory, or a combination of both. The P300 test is so named because the greatest brain response occurs at about 300 milliseconds after the stimulus.

A number of stimuli are presented to the patient (flashes or clicks, for example), and the computer records the responses. The response is assessed for its time (latency) and size (amplitude).

The QEP version of the test is performed with a full scalp of nineteen wires, so much more information is obtained. Naturally, this additional information is helpful to assess all parts of the brain, which are missed by the routine P300 test.

> ## QEP vs. traditional EP
>
> The QEP is superior to the traditional EP because it provides significantly more information, and thus all parts of the brain may be assessed. Many abnormalities may be seen and diagnosed with QEP that the routine EP does not assess, so the routine testing would miss the diagnosis (called false negatives) in a number of cases.

PATIENT CASE STUDY: COUP CONTRECOUP INJURY

Let's look at the case of Tom B., which shows the importance of using the most accurate testing methods available for diagnosing a TBI. Tom was wearing a seat belt as he drove his sporty coupe, which had worn rear tires, at the speed limit on a local highway. He was traveling north in the center lane and wanted to pass the car in front of him, which was moving at a much slower speed.

As Tom gently turned the wheel to the left to pass, the back tires of the coupe hit a puddle, and in a split second, his car suddenly turned hard to the left. He was unable to react in time, and his car went into the cement median at sixty miles per hour. The left front of the car struck the median, then the car bounced off and spun around three times before ending up in the service lane. The windows were blown out of the coupe.

When the car came to a stop, Tom saw that he had blood on his left arm. He did not know if he had hit his head, but he felt a lump forming on the back left side of his head. He was a little dazed and felt confused for a few minutes. He went to the local hospital and had a CT scan of his brain, which came back normal. He was discharged and sent home.

After the accident, Tom had neck pain, for which he went to therapy. After he finished the therapy, he began to notice that he was forgetful. He eventually came to my office, and I diagnosed him with post-concussion syndrome. He underwent a QEEG/QEP battery of tests, which confirmed the finding of a traumatic brain injury.

In the course of assessing Tom's work-up, I found two focal abnormalities, one in the left back of his brain and another in the right front. Most likely these were from hitting the back of his head on the left side on the headrest, causing his brain to slosh forward and to the right, which produced the right frontal focal area I saw in the abnormal testing. As described previously, this type of injury is called *coup contrecoup*. "Coup" refers to the site of the initial impact, and "contrecoup" (literally *backlash* in French) refers to the secondary injury.

Since Tom had such specific findings on his tests, I sent him for a MRI of his brain to rule out a structural lesion. A structural lesion is an injury that can be seen on an imaging scan, such as a CT or MRI scan, as opposed to a functional lesion, which can be detected only by a test such as a QEEG or SPECT scan. When the radiologist read the scan, she saw that there was indeed brain damage in the right front of Tom's brain. In fact, she called me and asked how I knew that there was a damaged area in the right front of the brain. I answered that both the QEEG and the QEP showed the damage.

The findings I saw on Tom's QEEG and QEP tests, however, were subtle on the standard EEG and easily missed. If the quantitative FFT and statistical analysis had not been done, these important findings would have been completely missed.

Tom's brain injury was moderate, and thus more severe than the typical mild traumatic brain injury (mTBI). The tests showed that he had suffered a classic coup contrecoup injury, when the brain is hit on one side and then the other side gets pushed up against the inner table at a diagonal to the initial injury. He was treated with a medication to increase blood flow in the brain, and made a partial recovery.

The cases presented in this chapter are from my actual practice in the 1990s. Over time, I added more patients to my study group, in which data from the QEEG and QEP were combined. I have determined that the most sensitive studies to document an mTBI remain the QEEG, the QEP, and the neuropsychological testing, followed by the SPECT scan, with the MRI being the least sensitive.

Modern diagnostic testing using SPECT, QEEG, and QEP provides much greater detail of TBIs, allowing for the detection of otherwise overlooked signs of concussion. They should be used in all cases of brain trauma to give accurate diagnoses. The tests should always be done with a normative database to ensure accuracy and not depend on anyone's opinion.

Until these sensitive instruments were developed, many concussions were never detected, leaving patients to suffer the effects of post-concussion syndrome with no resolution. Fortunately, now that we can detect such injuries, there are treatments that can and do heal them, leading to dramatically improved lives of thousands of patients. Part III goes into detail about the three powerful and proven methods I have used to successfully treat thousands of patients who sustained a traumatic brain injury.

Part III: Powerful Healing Solutions for Treating Concussions

Chapter 8

Method 1: Nimodipine

Traumatic brain injuries can happen to anyone at any time and for many reasons. The good news is that there are three proven methods of treating TBIs, all of which I have used for years with great success. I can state with certainty that my treatment works on anyone with a concussion, based on having treated thousands of patients with all types of brain injuries over the last few decades. All of my patients—from the most severely affected to the mildest—have responded to treatment.

In 1990, when I first began to order SPECT scans for many of my patients with TBI, I was impressed with what I saw in nearly all of them: they all had varying degrees of hypoperfusion, the reduced blood flow in the characteristic pattern described in chapter 7. I hypothesized that if essentially all patients had hypoperfusion, one treatment would be to increase the blood flow. Simple and elegant.

I was keenly aware of a specific FDA-approved medication for use in cases of bleeding in the brain of the subarachnoid hemorrhage (SAH) type, as discussed in chapter 2. This type of bleeding in the brain usually comes from an aneurysm that bursts, spilling blood throughout the area, but it can also be from trauma, when it is then called *traumatic subarachnoid hemorrage*, or tSAH.

In cases of tSAH, it has been established that bleeding in the brain causes a spasm of the brain's arteries. Recall from chapter 2 that this spasming causes hypoperfusion, ischemia (lack of oxygen), and sometimes complications such as stroke and seizures superimposed on the original injury.

The symptoms and signs in my patients ranged from the worst, such as paralysis and loss of language (aphasia), to milder ones, such as cognitive deficits, dizziness, and ringing of the ears (tinnitus, a difficult symptom to reverse through traditional methods). I concluded that in order to heal the brain, the treatment had to correct the underlying mechanism that caused the initial injury and the secondary dysfunction in the brain.

Indeed, my hypothesis turned out to be correct. When my patients took this particular medication, virtually all of them experienced improvement or total resolution of their symptoms.

NIMODIPINE

The first of the three methods I use to successfully treat traumatic brain injuries is a powerful drug called Nimotop (brand), or nimodipine (generic). Its official indication is for subarachnoid hemorrhage, but I prescribe it in an "off-label" manner. "Off label" simply means that a drug is prescribed for a condition that is not on the manufacturer's "label," or instructions, which doctors are allowed to do, and do so on a regular basis. In fact, some important discoveries have been made by prescribing medications off label, such as using Viagra, which was initially intended as a hypertension medication, for treating erectile dysfunction, a much larger market.

Both Nimotop and nimodipine, sometimes nicknamed "Nimo" by patients, are supplied in large 30 mg capsules. Ironically, the typical patients to whom this medication is prescribed are admitted to the intensive care unit (ICU) of a hospital and are often comatose, so they cannot swallow pills. In these instances, a nurse extracts the contents of the capsule with a needle and syringe, then administers it via a tube placed into the patient's stomach.

This is a tedious but necessary task, since the United States does not allow an intravenous or intramuscular route of administration, as do European countries (the medication was first introduced by Bayer Pharmaceutical, a German company). Therefore, for the most part, this medication is reserved for ICU use. I prescribe it for my patients, however, so I explain to them that the medication will have to be special ordered and that there will be a delay of a few days before they can pick it up at the pharmacy, as it is not kept in stock.

Safety and side effects of nimodipine

I have used nimodipine extensively to treat TBI and other neurological conditions in the outpatient setting with great success and safety. I have prescribed it to all age groups, from toddlers to octogenarians. Once a toddler took an adult dose by mistake, and afterward, his vital signs were regularly monitored while he continued to take the medication. He had no untoward side effects and actually benefited greatly, experiencing objective improvement of the hypoperfusion, which was documented on his post-treatment SPECT scan.

An adult patient once confused nimodipine with another medication that she had received from the pharmacy at the same time. She took many times the adult dose of the nimodipine on the first day, yet she did not feel any bad side effects. When she came back to see me, I advised her to obtain a cardiac consult as a safety precaution, which she did. It proved to be completely normal.

These examples are recounted to demonstrate the safety of nimodipine. When I prescribe the drug, I always start with a low dose, such as one capsule three times a day, and instruct patients to look for side effects as well as benefits. I ask them to return for follow-up on a monthly basis, and if there are no problems at each visit with the current dosage, I increase it upward.

The maximum dosage I have prescribed was five capsules (a total of 150 mg) three times a day, or 450 mg a day. In that case, which was a severe TBI with gross bleeding in the brain and complicated by an initial coma of several months, the patient developed the side effect of peripheral edema (fluid retention in the extremities, usually the legs), but it was a trade-off. The patient showed improved neurological function while enduring the edema. This case is presented in case study 1 in chapter 13.

Regarding side effects, I have observed, and only on high doses, patients experience peripheral edema in the lower legs. In only one case did I see very mild edema in the legs and hands of a patient who had suffered a stroke (CVA, or cerebrovascular accident) and had residual numbness on one side of his body. He took the standard dose of the medication for about two months, after which time he did not want to tolerate the edema any longer. Nevertheless, most of his residual numbness resolved.

HOW NIMODIPINE HEALS THE BRAIN

Certainly at this point, it is logical to inquire about how nimodipine works. This medication is in the class of drugs known as calcium channel blockers. However, this type of calcium blocker is different from the others in that it is specific to the cerebral arteries in the brain.

Nimodipine is very liposoluble, meaning it can dissolve in fatty substances, permitting it to penetrate through the blood-brain barrier (BBB) and into the brain. The BBB is a protective mechanism that keeps unwanted substances from entering the brain.

Calcium channel blockers

A calcium channel blocker works by closing the calcium channel, or receptor, on the surface of an artery or any vessel carrying oxygenated blood in the brain. Closing, or blocking, the calcium channel prevents calcium from getting into the cell, thus preventing the cascade of metabolic events within the cells that culminates in cell death (apoptosis), as discussed in chapter 2.

It also relaxes the smooth muscles inside the artery, which facilitates the artery's dilatation. This, in turn, increases blood flow, so more oxygen is delivered to the cell. The drug was not designed to act on any arteries outside of the brain, as other members in this class of medications do, which explains why there are so few systemic side effects.

Research on nimodipine

In 1990, when I first started to prescribe nimodipine, I felt as though I were a pioneer embarking on a new path in order to provide a treatment that was very much needed. Perhaps other practitioners were doing the same as I was, but if they were, I didn't know about it, and I never published my data, since I was not in an academic environment.

Clearly, scientific studies with properly designed controlled studies using nimodipine for mTBIs are needed and should be performed. The biggest obstacle to this research is finding an entity that would finance the expense of a clinical trial. If a new patent for nimodipine could be obtained for a new indication (there is only one indication now, for subarachnoid hemorrhage), there may be a chance that a pharmaceutical company would finance the study.

Nimodipine has been available as a generic drug for a number of years. I would like to find a pharmaceutical company that would be interested in funding a clinical trial of nimodipine for mTBI. Such a trial is greatly needed to prove the efficacy of the drug for this condition.

NYMALIZE: A NEW DOSING FORM

In 2018, after I had been prescribing nimodipine for twenty-eight years, I discovered another form of nimodipine. The brand name Nymalize is nimodipine in liquid form, and comes in two different strengths: the standard 30 mg in 10 ml of fluid and 60 mg in 20 ml of fluid. It was approved by the FDA in May 2013 as the first oral solution of nimodipine, so it is currently available only as a brand medication.

Having a liquid form of this medication is advantageous for hospital patients, since in the original large capsule form, nurses had to extract the contents with a syringe and then push the medication down a tube to get it into the stomach of the unconscious patient, as previously explained. It also makes a difference for outpatients and children who are unable to swallow the large pill.

WHY NIMODIPINE?

As you have read here and will read more of in the case studies in chapter 13, nimodipine works very well to supply blood to the areas of the brain with hypoperfusion, thus leading to improvements, often dramatic. I strongly advocate for its use in most if not all TBIs, as its remarkable benefits are undeniable.

Among the three proven methods to treat concussion, patients most often choose to take the medication as the choice of treatment, because if the patient has insurance to cover the prescription, then they can always get the medication. In many instances, a patient may not be able to afford to pay out of pocket for the other proven methods of neurofeedback and hyperbaric oxygen because they are typically not covered by insurance and are somewhat expensive.

Nimodipine is just one of these three proven methods and is incredibly effective. It is easy to take, and improvements may be seen in a short amount of time. When combined with the other two methods, patients will most likely experience quite noticeable improvements of symptoms, including the ability to walk and talk where they couldn't before treatment.

Chapter 9

Method 2: Neurofeedback Therapy

Neurofeedback is a specific treatment modality that retrains the brain by taking advantage of the brain's *neuroplasticity*, the ability of the brain to create new connections between neurons after an injury. Neurofeedback (NFB) changes the brain's electrical function by using positive reinforcement through repeated sessions. NFB converts the dysfunctional state of the brain into a more normal state, as determined by a normative database.

Neurofeedback, the second of the three powerful methods I use to treat TBI, is similar to biofeedback but is applied to the brain. Most people are familiar with the term *biofeedback*, which is a procedure that retrains various bodily functions.

BIOFEEDBACK

To perform a biofeedback session, a sensor attached to the biofeedback instrument is placed on a part of the person's body, where the sensor measures, for example, skin temperature or pulse. The person is asked to relax or to perform a simple task such as concentrating on something. If they perform the action as requested, they get a reward of some kind, thus reinforcing the behavior.

For example, say a person wants to learn a method to reduce their stress. They are seated in a comfortable chair, and a sensor is attached to one of their fingertips. They are given specific instructions on how to relax, and at the same time, they look at a computer screen that displays a reading of their pulse. As they relax, their pulse slows, indicating a correct response. They can see the desired change in their pulse rate, which is the reward, on the screen. As the person continues to look at the computer screen, their mental effort at relaxing reinforces the ongoing response of a slower pulse.

The visual input from the computer screen sustains the continuous cycle of relax-reward. This circular nature gives biofeedback its name. *Bio* refers to the fact that a specific biological function is monitored and modified if the person performs correctly. There are many biological functions that can be used in addition to skin temperature and pulse, such as muscle tension and spasm. When sensors are placed on the scalp, biofeedback may be used for a headache.

Most types of biofeedback involve the relaxation of blood vessels to increase blood flow, increase the temperature of the hands, or relax muscles to reduce pain.

The history of biofeedback

The origin of biofeedback and thus neurofeedback may be traced back millennia, to the origins of yoga and meditation, although the term biofeedback was not coined until 1969. The original research on biofeedback was conducted in the 1930s by Edmund Jacobsen, and then by Johanne Schultz. Sometimes biofeedback is called "the yoga of the west," since the same physiological principles apply. What biofeedback and yoga have in common is the ability of the mind to interact with the body in specific patterns.

Various biofeedback techniques were developed in the 1960s, with the original work conducted on animals. At first, researchers experimented with controlling blood pressure, muscle function, and heart function. One investigator, scientist and psychologist Joe Kamiya, studied perception and how it could be manipulated. He discovered that certain individuals could control their own brain waves and even learn how to produce specific brain waves on demand.

At the Menninger Institute in Houston, Texas, where different types of feedback were studied, one volunteer used skin temperature techniques to abort a migraine headache. All of these methods, when applied to the brain by placing sensors on the scalp, formed the basis of what became known as neurofeedback (NFB).

THE DEVELOPMENT OF NEUROFEEDBACK

Berger discovered alpha waves in the 1950s and Kamiya was the first to use biofeedback on the alpha brain wave in the awake-and-alert state. In the 1970s, psychologist and neuroscientist Barry Sterman found he could suppress epileptic seizures in cats, and later, in humans. Sterman was also the first to discover that the brain could be modified in function and structure, a concept only recently termed *neuroplasticity*.

Psychologist and researcher (and a consultant to parts of this book) Joel F. Lubar found he could treat attention-deficit hyperactivity disorder (ADHD) and hyperactivity with NFB. In the early 2000s, the American Association of Psychologists awarded NFB with the highest level of psychosocial intervention for treatment of attention deficit and hyperactivity. In the 1980s, psychologist Eugene O. Peniston treated alcoholic Vietnam War veterans with neurofeedback techniques.

In the early days of neurofeedback, the equipment and computers used to perform the treatments were primitive, bulky, slow, and expensive, which meant that NFB therapy was restricted to universities. With the advent of smaller and faster computers, private doctors could afford to purchase the necessary equipment and train to perform NFB.

Initially, NFB was conducted with two to four sensors placed on the scalp in specific areas. The placement of the sensors was either standardized or customized to specific areas that were read as abnormal on a patient's EEG. The subject was hooked up to the sensors, which were attached to a computer, and the therapist would ask the subject to perform a task. Subjects could, for example, play a game or listen to music, as long as they attended to the task.

When a subject succeeded in performing the task, a reward was generated, which in turn corrected the existing abnormal brain waves. This type of treatment is called *surface neurofeedback*. Other practitioners developed their own protocols, such as starting the treatment in one quadrant of the brain and then proceeding to an adjacent quadrant, moving counterclockwise around the head.

QEEG AND NFB

Before NFB is initiated, a thorough interview of the patient as well as a proper QEEG should be conducted. There are practitioners who will treat without performing a QEEG, but I think this practice is not prudent and may even be dangerous, because if there is no baseline of abnormal brain waves, then the practitioner would not know where to start treatment. When the QEEG is performed correctly and shows specific brain wave abnormalities, then a treatment protocol can be developed that is specific for that particular individual.

As with all other methods of treatment, NFB has evolved thanks to advances of technology and software. Recall the LORETA test (chapter 7), which provides information as images of slices of the brain, where the information represents the electrical activity of the brain. This is an important test because many surface abnormalities that are seen on the plain EEG come from sources that are deeper in the brain, and only the LORETA method can disclose them at those depths.

One of the reasons to diagnose these deeper lesions is that when these sites are treated directly, they can be corrected more quickly and efficiently than by surface neurofeedback alone. Recall also that when the QEEG is performed, a statistical analysis of a particular abnormality is also performed, which determines how abnormal the particular problem is. This technique is applied to the LORETA slices so that we can see how abnormal the findings are.

ADVANCEMENT IN NFB

A major advance in NFB occurred when the technology was developed that enabled feedback from an entire set of nineteen sensors on the scalp (as with recording an EEG). There are many advantages to performing NFB with a full set of sensors on the scalp.

First, the entire brain can be treated instead of just one part or lobe. Second, new software has allowed us to target the deep sources of abnormalities. When these abnormalities are treated directly, they can be corrected faster and more thoroughly. Treatment time can be cut in half because of the much higher efficacy of the treatment.

Some conditions were difficult to treat before LORETA-type feedback because the source of the problem emanated from deep centers of the brain and were not amenable to treatment by the surface method. A good example of this is post-traumatic stress disorder, which is so common in veterans returning from the wars in Iraq and Afghanistan.

The last point to make about the advantages of LORETA neurofeedback over other types, especially surface NFB, is that it should always be performed with a statistical analysis, which is called *Z-Score LORETA NFB*. Recall that when the QEEG is performed, each aspect that is tested is evaluated by statistical analysis, so the most accurate type of NFB should always be performed with a simultaneous Z score. The reason is obvious: the practitioner needs to know if the results are normal or not, and if not, how abnormal they are.

The Z-score LORETA neurofeedback

To perform a typical Z-score LORETA NFB, the patient is seated comfortably in a chair. A cap is used to place the sensors on the scalp, the instrument is calibrated, and the brain training begins.

As previously mentioned, the stimulus for the patient may be, for example, watching a movie or playing a game, which young adults and children prefer. If the person watches the movie or plays the video game with an honest effort, the effort expended is the actual reward. The reward in turn repairs the brain damage by producing new normal brain wave patterns.

Each session lasts about fifty minutes, which is divided into several rounds of five to ten minutes each. The training is typically done twice a week but may be up to twice a day. Most diligent therapists will reassess the Z score after each session to ensure that the treatment is beneficial.

After one week of treatment, a trend analysis is produced in graph form. This shows if the trend of the Z score is decreasing (or increasing, if the starting Z score is negative). The eventual goal is to lower (or raise) the score to a normal level. When the goal is attained, the treatment should be stopped so as to not overtreat. Overtreating a patient, which can happen if the therapist does not use the Z-score method to monitor improvements, can cause harm. It is easily avoided by using the Z-score analysis method.

After the NFB therapy is completed, a post-treatment QEEG should be performed to ensure that all pre-treatment abnormalities are gone. Sometimes, and especially in complicated cases, new abnormalities are revealed by the post-treatment QEEG, and in these cases, another round of NFB should be instituted. (For those interested in learning more about this powerful technique to repair and fix your brain, please consult the textbook *Z-Score LORETA Neurofeedback: Clinical Applications* [Robert Thatcher and Joel Lubar, eds., Waltham, MA: Academic Press, 2014]. I had the honor of contributing a chapter, co-written with my colleague Gerald Gluck, PhD, called "LORETA and SPECT Scans: A Correlational Case Series," in which we demonstrated for the first time that there was a positive correlation of findings of the two diagnostic tests between 90 and 100 percent of the time.)

I recall one patient who had a concussion and received NFB for several years. In the beginning, he could not stay awake during the treatment sessions and required a stimulant medication. After several years, he had improved to the point at which he no longer needed the stimulant, and he felt that he had made a full recovery. His moving story is included at the end of this chapter.

I recall another patient who had NFB for many years and continued to show gradual improvement. His problem was a seizure disorder with an underlying abnormal brain structure that predisposed him to having seizures. As his treatments progressed and various abnormalities were resolved, new ones showed up on post-treatment QEEG tests, necessitating further NFB sessions. The continued treatments, combined with a seizure medication, resulted in successfully eradicating his auras and eliminating his seizures.

THE BEST APPROACH TO NFB THERAPY

Neurofeedback therapy should always start with a properly performed QEEG. It should also include a LORETA analysis and statistical comparison of the individual with a group of his or her peers. The LORETA should always be performed with a full scalp of nineteen electrodes, and a Z-score analysis should be performed after treatment.

When seeking out a neurofeedback therapist, always ask if the practitioner performs or has someone else perform a baseline QEEG, because the QEEG is the most accurate and effective method of evaluating the brain's electrical function. Also ask if they use LORETA Z-score training, because LORETA NFB is the most effective and fastest type of NFB therapy to correct abnormal brain waves. If they do not use these state-of-the-art treatment modalities, my recommendation is to find another provider, even if you have to travel a distance. It will be worth it.

A Patient's Endorsement

I was in a broadside auto collision in March 2016 and suffered a severe concussion and traumatic brain injury. I saw Dr. Gerald Gluck, one of the world's leading experts in the field of neurofeedback, who referred me to Dr. Wand. After seeing both of these gifted doctors, I went from literally being barely able to function to now being close to normal.

Dr. Wand's integrative approach drew on the best of all approaches to healing. These included conventional allopathic medicine, an out-of-the-box prescription pharmaceutical medication [nimodipine], vitamins and truly cutting-edge herbal supplements, spectral analysis [from FFT], acupuncture, massage, ultrasound, hyperbaric oxygen therapy, and the jewel of his medical toolbox, LORETA neurofeedback. Also, Dr. Wand's extraordinary scope of knowledge as both a neurologist and a diagnostician cannot be overstated.

Dr. Wand is an integrative neurologist who seeks what every field of medicine can best offer his patients. Nothing he recommends escapes his scrutiny, personal research, and keen mind. When a claim is made, he personally tests and re-tests the hypothesis in consultation with his esteemed cadre of medical colleagues before he will recommend what might otherwise seem unconventional or alternative to his patients.

I strongly recommend Dr. Wand, a true healing innovator steeped in the rich tradition of what traditional medical doctors have to offer, and who is also unabashedly passionate about integrating the best of what complimentary medicine contributes to the spectrum of healing.

—Mark Knobel

The brain has the extraordinary ability to develop new connections between neurons, known as neuroplasticity. This remarkable ability can be exploited by actively engaging in brain-wave training through the proven method of neurofeedback.

When combined with the other methods discussed in Part III, patients may experience a full recovery after a traumatic brain injury. Chapter 10 explores the third and final method for treating a TBI, rounding out the successful protocol I have used with my patients with tremendous success for many years.

Chapter 10

Method 3: Hyperbaric Oxygen Therapy

Hyperbaric oxygen therapy, or HBOT, is a treatment that pumps pure oxygen into the blood. The normal air that we breathe contains 20 percent oxygen, but HBOT air is 100 percent oxygen, and thus delivers five times more oxygen to the cells. HBOT is the third of the three powerful methods I use to treat traumatic brain injuries.

The benefits of using HBOT include its unique ability to heal any kind of wound, which means it is beneficial for treating brain injuries in TBI patients. When all factors are considered, the single most important criterion to effect healing is making oxygen available to the cells of the body, for without sufficient oxygen, cells simply cannot heal or function properly.

HBOT is probably best known for its ability to heal wounds when all other measures fail. It is, in fact, so well established in the medical field that practically all insurance will pay for its services for most wound healing, especially since it is cheaper than paying for a mutilating surgery such as amputation. Unfortunately, however, treatment for the brain is not generally covered. HBOT is also well known as the treatment of choice when scuba divers ascend too rapidly and develop a condition called the bends, in which nitrogen builds up in the blood. HBOT helps to dissolve the nitrogen bubbles.

The common denominator in all of these conditions, and in any condition that requires healing, is the need for additional oxygen to promote and allow healing. Quite simply, oxygen is king.

HBOT vs. ambient air

The difference between an ordinary oxygen treatment and hyperbaric oxygen is that ordinary oxygen treatment is given at ambient air pressure at various percentages of oxygen, while in an HBOT treatment, 100 percent pure oxygen is pumped into a closed, airtight chamber at varying pressures.

Ambient air, the normal air that we breathe, is equal to one atmosphere of pressure, or ATM. When either air or pure oxygen is compressed in an airtight chamber, the ATM of each increases. Typical pressures used to treat various conditions range from 1.2 to 2.0 ATM.

To commence an HBOT treatment, the patient is placed inside the chamber, then the pressure is gradually increased to reach the desired level. The patient inhales the pressurized pure oxygen for the prescribed time. When the time is up, the pressure is slowly decreased, and the treatment is complete.

The start-up and the slow-down of pressure adds to the total treatment time, which is typically ninety minutes. About sixty minutes of that is actual treatment time.

A LITERATURE REVIEW

When doctors and other professionals want to see the results of their colleagues' research, they conduct what is called a literature review. This helps provide them with an overview of the research results and may guide them in their own treatments. It is a common method of learning and keeping up with the newest findings and up-to-date treatments.

I conducted a review of the literature on HBOT for mTBI. Interestingly, there was not a lot of research in this area, but I did find one small study that evaluated fifty-six patients. The study was conducted in a scientific manner such that the results are considered valid.

The patients were all diagnosed with TBI that had occurred from between one and five years prior to the study, which means that they had already improved by whatever treatment they had undergone and through the innate ability of the brain and body to heal. The patients were tested before treatment with a SPECT scan and some cognitive tests. They had all had the usual forty treatments of HBOT. They were all re-tested after treatment to assess for any improvement. Every single patient showed improvement, and in fact, the post-treatment SPECT scan demonstrated a relative increase of 27 percent blood flow. This result is remarkable.

I found one other small study of twenty-nine veterans who were injured in the wars in the Middle East. The design of this study was similar to the one just described. One difference was that the vets were evaluated for PTSD, a signature injury of the Iraq and Afghanistan wars and known to be difficult to treat. The article concluded that all conditions, including PTSD, improved after treatment, not only after just one day of treatment but also six months after the treatment ended. In addition, SPECT scans performed six months after treatment showed that 75 percent of the areas in the brain that had been abnormal had reverted to normal. The conclusion was that HBOT was considered to be safe and effective for this type of treatment.

HOW HBOT HELPS TO HEAL THE BRAIN

There are many explanations for how HBOT promotes the healing of any tissue, but this discussion will address only how the therapy works to heal the brain. As previously mentioned, oxygen is the single most important element for the healing of human tissues.

When the diameter of a blood vessel in the brain narrows because of a TBI, the blood flow through it decreases, and stops altogether if the vessel completely closes. When this happens, the oxygen level falls, and then all of the tissues downstream from the point of closure suffer the inevitable fate of dying unless the blood flow is restored. The end result is ischemia (lack of oxygen) and apoptosis (cell death), as explained in chapter 2. Recall from chapter 8 that the medication nimodipine increases blood flow and thus increases the oxygen level to the tissues, promoting healing.

The first and most obvious way in which HBOT promotes healing is that it increases the oxygen level in the circulating blood via the respiratory system as the patient simply breaths the enriched air that fills the chamber. Also, since the air is pressurized, the oxygen can pass directly through the skin and into all of the tissues, including the vascular system, and thereby improve all bodily functions.

Even though HBOT is known to oxygenate the tissues in the brain and facilitate healing, it is rarely used for treating TBI. While HBOT is known as a last resort treatment to heal most wounds and injuries and is covered by most insurance, this is not the case for treating concussion. To learn more about why HBOT is underutilized as a treatment for TBI, please see appendix B.

HBOT AND INFLAMMATION

Whenever the body sustains an injury, it responds with inflammation, which then induces an anti-inflammatory response. For example, if you step barefoot on a thorn, the site of the injury immediately hurts, calling your attention to it and pushing you to remove the cause of the pain. This is followed by secondary symptoms such as swelling, inflammation, and bruising with bleeding under the skin. These symptoms persist until the body's healing mechanisms take over. Once this happens, the body absorbs the blood and its by-products, reducing the swelling and bruising.

There are many chemicals involved in the process of creating inflammation, which explains why doctors often prescribe medications such as anti-inflammatories to suppress the symptoms that occur from the inflammation. While inflammation is in fact the body's natural response to an injury and serves an important role in healing, it can also prevent healing if it persists for too long.

Like any other damaged organ in the body, the brain responds to an injury with inflammation, swelling, and bleeding, but the consequences are quite different, since the functions of the brain are unique and unlike those of other parts of the body.

Many studies have shown that HBOT can reduce inflammation in the brain. The overall conclusion from these studies was that hyperbaric oxygen therapy for TBI is associated with improving the neurological outcome and reducing swelling in the brain, leakage of the blood-brain barrier, and cell apoptosis.

HBOT AND APOPTOSIS

Apoptosis is the destruction of a cell that results in the cell's death. It is part of the normal life cycle of any cell, but it is meant to happen only at a designated time based on the cell's natural lifespan.

However, cells may be injured or damaged in numerous ways. Two of the most common are traumatic brain injury and stroke. In the case of TBI, neurons begin to die within hours after the injury, and secondary effects, called *secondary injuries*, may last for weeks or longer. In the area surrounding the main site of the injury, a second population of neurons are injured but alive. Targeting these cells for treatment is important because their injury is reversible, so it is possible to heal them and return their function back to normal.

HBOT AND INTRACRANIAL HYPERTENSION

The cerebrospinal fluid (CSF) is distributed throughout the brain, sent down into the spinal cord, and then pumped back up to the brain, creating a continuous circuit. If this circuit is blocked, the CSF can build up and cause an increase of pressure called *intracranial hypertension*, or ICP, which can cause brain damage.

The pressure of the CSF can also increase when the contents of the brain increase. This can happen from a mass such as a tumor or blood clot. When this happens, the volume of the brain itself increases from swelling, which can further increase the ICP.

Recall from chapter 2 that when the brain expands, it pushes the underlying brain deeper down, literally squashing the lower brain. When this pressure is great enough in an acute TBI, swelling develops, contributing even more damage and leading to ICP. In fact, ICP is a leading cause of increased illness and death in severe TBI.

HBOT has the ability to reduce ICP by increasing oxygen to the damaged tissue, thereby reducing the swelling and promoting the healing of injured cells.

HBOT, ANGIOGENESIS, AND NEUROGENESIS

Angiogenesis refers to the formation of new blood vessels. An example is a growing child, in whom all parts of the body increase in size and number, including the blood vessels. Another less obvious example is cancer, where there is a wild increase in the numbers of cells and vessels that require extra blood flow to satisfy the needs of the cancerous cells.

In animal studies, test subjects with concussion were treated with HBOT. When their brains were analyzed, the data showed favorable responses from the HBOT treatment. Researchers found reduced inflammation, angiogenesis, newly formed neurons (*neurogenesis*), and an increase of supporting cells to the neurons. There was also evidence of new connections between neurons called *synapses*, which helped the animals' motor abilities.

One HBOT human study showed significant improvement of blood flow and volume in the brain and improved results in psychological testing. These included an increase in the speed of thinking, which is always slowed when a brain injury occurs. SPECT scans were used to document blood flow before and after treatment. The post-treatment scans visually showed a significant increase of blood flow in those areas that had showed significant hypoperfusion.

The authors of this elegant study were able to document for the first time in humans suffering from persistent post-concussion symptoms (PPCS) that HBOT could induce healing months or even years after an injury. (This matches my observations using nimodipine.) They also found improved angiogenesis and an increase in neuroplasticity, which assists in cellular repair and clinical recovery, even years after the injury.

In summary, there are three proven methods that address and correct what goes wrong in the brain after a concussion and that I have used with great success for many years. While each individual method can reverse the symptoms of a concussion, I have repeatedly observed that when two of the methods—or even better, all three—are administered together, the improvement is increased, often dramatically. The effect of combined therapies being greater than the results of each individual effect is referred to as a *synergistic effect.*

There are other therapies that complement the nimodipine, neurofeedback, and hyperbaric oxygen therapy treatments. The next chapter addresses a supplement therapy I recommend that may be used in combination with the three proven methods to treat concussion. It also discusses a treatment that should always be undertaken when TBI affects hormone levels in the body.

Chapter 11

Natural Supplements Therapy

In chapter 8 we looked at treating TBI with the pharmaceutical drug nimodipine, an FDA-approved calcium channel blocker. In this chapter we will discuss an alternative choice of natural substances, also called *nutraceuticals*.

My approach for recommending supplements is based on the neuroanatomy and neurophysiology of the brain's neurons. Many supplements can help to heal brain injuries and benefit the brain in general by supporting the healing of damaged neurons. It helps to have some understanding of the structure of neurons.

THE STRUCTURE OF NEURONS

The two main components of a neuron are the cell body and its connections, including an axon (nerve fiber) that sends information away from the cell body, and dendrites (extensions of the nerve cell), which bring information to the cell body.

These cellular components have the cell membrane in common. The structure is complex but well known. In general terms, the cell membrane has a double layer of fat-soluble biochemicals made primarily of omega fatty acids, in particular EPA and DHA. Since these two omega 3s are considered main building blocks of the cell membrane, it is logical for people to consume appropriate amounts of these healthy fatty acids to ensure proper maintenance of existing membranes, and to aid in the development of newly forming neurons.

Another important component of the cell membrane is called *phosphatidylserine*, a fatty substance that enables the membrane to remain fluid and assists in the conduction of nerve impulses. Membrane function can be enhanced by eating more *choline alfoscerate*, or alpha GPC, which works by acting as a precursor to the fatty layer in cell membranes. Alpha GPC is available in supplement form.

Brain cells communicate via specialized chemicals called *neurotransmitters*. These vital chemicals are released from a structure in the membrane, cross the tiny space between the neurons, and are caught by structure on the receiving neuron.

Neurotransmitters, made inside the neurons, require precursors, or building blocks, to be synthesized, so it makes sense to provide these building blocks for each of type of transmitter. The most common neurotransmitters include the compound *acetylcholine* (known to decrease in Alzheimer's disease), *serotonin* (found to decrease in different types of depression), GABA (an amino acid), and dopamine (involved with reward and pleasure, and known to be deficient in Parkinson's disease). For each of these transmitters, there are specific supplements, such as CDP-choline, that aid in their synthesis.

The lack of regulation of nutraceuticals

While the US Food and Drug Administration (FDA) is federally mandated to protect the public by ensuring the safety and efficacy of approved drugs, there is no analogous organization charged with the supervision of nutraceuticals. It follows that quality control in the industry may be lacking.

The only way to trust a manufacturer of vitamins and supplements is to see a document called a certificate of analysis (COA). This certificate is a laboratory document that describes the analysis of the raw product used to make a vitamin or supplement.

Each manufacturer should have analyses performed by two or three neutral, independent laboratories before, during, and after manufacture. Some manufacturers, however, perform their own analyses "in house," which is not considered ethical because of an inherent bias that cannot be ruled out.

Analysis by independent laboratories has been fully espoused by Life Extension® (www.lifeextension.com), a premier privately owned antiaging company headquartered in Fort Lauderdale, Florida. I have had the opportunity to review many COAs of the raw products the company uses to make their vitamins and supplements. I was quite impressed with the purity of these raw products, which are typically rated at greater than 90 percent purity. Life Extension makes COAs readily available upon request.

All of the supplements recommended in this chapter are available through the Life Extension website.

VITAMINS AND SUPPLEMENTS FOR TBI

There are many excellent vitamins and supplements available that support the healing of damaged neurons, reduce hypoperfusion, and help the brain heal in other ways. This section describes several of them and explains how they provide support for TBI.

Ginkgo biloba

The loss of blood flow, or hypoperfusion, that occurs in a TBI and that I consider to be the hallmark injury in concussion can be combatted with supplements. Many supplements are thought to increase blood flow in the brain if they are able to pass through the BBB, which enables them to act directly within the cells.

Probably the most well known of these is Ginkgo biloba, which comes from one of the oldest known tree species. Ginkgo biloba has many health benefits. It supports healthy circulation, helps to maintain the normal function and tone of blood vessels, supports healthy oxygen and glucose metabolism in the brain, stabilizes capillaries and makes them less fragile, supports normal blood coagulation, and supports healthy aging in the brain.

Ginkgo leaf extract contains several active components, including flavonoids, terpenes, lactones, and organic acids, all of which have neuroprotective and cardioprotective properties. Flavonoids, phytonutrients found in most fruits and vegetables, are especially important, as they are powerful antioxidants. They also protect the mitochondria, the "powerhouses" inside cells that produce oxygen and energy for the entire body. Mitochondria are vital to how well the cells function.

When choosing a Ginkgo biloba supplement, purity is vital because the raw plant contains a chemical called ginkgolic acid, a relative of poison ivy. Look for a label stating that the product does not contain more than 5 ppm of ginkgolic acid.

Any Ginkgo biloba product you choose should also be at least a 24 percent extract and have at least 6 percent terpene lactones. If these percentages are not listed on the label, I suggest that you continue searching for a product that meets these standards.

PQQ

A supplement called PQQ increases oxygen within the cell via a completely unique ability: it increases the number of mitochondria inside the cell. Scientific research has documented that PQQ enters the mitochondria within the cell and induces it to replicate through a process is called *mitochondrial biogenesis.*

All mitochondria possess their own DNA independent of the nuclear DNA, but this DNA is less protected than the DNA in the nucleus. As a result, the DNA inside mitochondria are more subject to oxidative stress. PQQ (pyrroloquinoline quinone) works as an antioxidant to protect the mitochondrial DNA.

When it is taken in capsule form, PQQ is distributed throughout the entire body and is therefore beneficial to all organs, especially those with high metabolic demand, such as the brain and the heart. In fact, modern theories of aging are recognizing more pathologies related to mitochondrial dysfunction. Supplementing with PQQ is a recommended treatment.

Since anti-aging philosophy promotes applying preventive methods *before* irreversible damage occurs in the body, its products are designed to address specific issues such as mitochondrial dysfunction. The recommended dose is 20 mg of PQQ, preferably taken before food.

CoQ10

Research has shown that PQQ works well with another supplement called CoQ10. This antioxidant is a vital co-factor in the Krebs cycle, the biochemical pathway that makes oxygen from glucose and energy for the body.

NATURAL ANTI-INFLAMMATORY SUPPLEMENTS

Anti-inflammatory supplements can help reduce inflammation in the brain after a traumatic injury. It is important to choose supplements that pass through the BBB and provide anti-inflammatory action. The body always responds to a trauma with inflammation, but excessive inflammation can inhibit the healing process, hence the importance of taking the correct anti-inflammatory products.

There are several types of anti-inflammatory supplements that have little or no side effects, whereas some pharmaceuticals can have severe side effects. Several pharmaceuticals of non-steroidal anti-inflammatories (NSAIDS) class pass through the BBB but have significant side effects, which precludes their long-term use. Newer evidence suggests that even the short-term use of NSAIDS may have harmful side effects. Supplements do not have such adverse side effects and can be recommended for long-term use.

Curcumin

Probably the most well-known natural anti-inflammatory is curcumin, the active ingredient in an Indian spice called turmeric. Curcumin is a type of root called a rhizome that contains polyphenols, micronutrients with many health benefits. Interestingly, epidemiological data suggests that the incidence of Alzheimer's-type dementia occurs less frequently in India compared to other countries. Curry, which contains curcumin, is a popular spice in India and is added to many foods.

Curcumin also has clinical benefits as a systemic anti-inflammatory, so it can be taken on a regular basis without worry of ulcers, heart attack, and other side effects associated with NSAIDS.

Boswellia serrata

You may have heard of NSAIDS that are named after the inflammatory pathways of COX 1 and COX 2, but we rarely hear about the *lipoxygenase pathway*, or LOX. This pathway becomes more active from poor diet, especially with the consumption of omega 6-FFA (free fatty acid). Aging may be associated with increased 5 LOX activity, leading to the increased production of *leukotriene B4*. This pro-inflammatory mediator breaks down the LOX into a metabolite that attacks various body parts, such as joints and arterial walls.

Fortunately, there is a natural substance that can neutralize 5 LOX. It comes from an Indian plant called *Boswellia serrata*. Based on animal studies, this substance, which is a 5-LOX inhibitor, passes through the blood-brain barrier, where it can have a beneficial effect on the brain.

Omega 3 fatty acids

One particular supplement deserves special mention, since it is very important to one's general health, and specifically to brain health. It is omega 3 fatty acids, which are essential to maintain neuronal cell membrane health.

The process to manufacture this supplement is complex and requires specialized equipment that can perform molecular distillation to produce the purest product. To maintain the highest standard of the manufacture of omega 3 fatty acids, all manufacturers should have their products tested rigorously by an organization called the International Fish Oil Standards (IFOS).[1]

Magnesium

Magnesium is a mineral that plays many critical roles in the body and is crucial to hundreds of enzymes that perform vital functions. It plays a key role in relaxing the arteries in the brain that go into spasm after a trauma.[2]

Magnesium enters the wall of the artery in a site called a calcium receptor. When the magnesium is in the proper place in the receptor, its action prevents the spasming of the artery, thereby preventing hypoperfusion and secondary ischemia. Because of this protection, magnesium is said to be *neuroprotective*. The role of calcium channel blocking agents is vital to the mechanism of restoring blood flow, which is how the brain heals.

Up to 80 percent of the US population is deficient in magnesium and is unaware of it. Many people suffer from common conditions such as leg cramps, hypertension, and migraine headaches because of a lack of magnesium.

The full value of magnesium is often overlooked by allopathic medicine, where it is primarily used to treat eclampsia, a complication of pregnancy consisting of fluid retention, hypertension, and seizures. Interestingly, when patients with eclampsia arrive at the hospital while having seizures, including non-stop seizures usually resistant to standard treatment, they are not administered anti-epilepsy drugs. Instead, they are given intravenous magnesium sulfate, which is quite successful in treating all of these symptoms.

---

[1] The interested reader can read "Relentless Commitment to Quality," which is a detailed analysis published by Life Extension in 2015. See https://www.lifeextension.com/Magazine/2015/7/Relentless-Commitment-To-Quality/Page-01.
[2] See *The Magnesium Miracle* by Carolyn Dean for more information on the importance of magnesium.

The miracle of magnesium

There is abundant information on the clinical effects of magnesium in humans. Most of the pertinent research information on magnesium is reviewed in *The Magnesium Miracle*, an excellent book by Carolyn Dean, MD, ND. I highly recommend the book, as it has so much good information about this precious mineral.

Magnesium is underrated and underappreciated in its role in the human body. In my own case, I was having a problem controlling my hypertension despite taking two different classes of anti-hypertensive medication, to which I had to add a diuretic to achieve somewhat better control. Since I have been taking a product developed by Dr. Dean, my blood pressure is steadily going down, and it is already lower than when I was taking the pharmaceuticals alone.

Throughout her book, Dr. Dean emphasizes that magnesium is neuroprotective, prevents strokes, treats migraines and other non-neurological conditions associated with smooth-muscle spasms such as asthma with wheezing, and decreases or prevents spasms of the arteries, which in turn helps to treat TBI.

Studies have shown that when a TBI is sustained, the magnesium level in the blood plasma fall dramatically. After an acute TBI, the calcium level in the blood increases, competing with the magnesium, causing the magnesium to decrease even more. This competition contributes to a cascade of events that lead to apoptosis, or cell death, as described in chapter 2.

There is an inverse relationship between the level of magnesium and the severity of the TBI such that the more severe the TBI, the lower the magnesium level. Conversely, the higher the magnesium level is, the better the outcome and recovery from TBI. Clinical research using intravenous magnesium after TBI has shown improved cognitive functioning.

Stroke and magnesium

A brief discussion is in order regarding stroke and magnesium, since the common denominator with TBI is the vascular connection. Epidemiological data has shown that higher levels of magnesium in drinking water are associated with lower incidents of stroke. One study showed that lower dietary magnesium was associated with higher risk of hypertension and stroke.

Many years of research have shown that reducing the serum magnesium level is associated with spasming of the arteries, whereas increasing its level is associated with relaxing the arteries. Magnesium also serves a critical function as a co-factor in the calcium channel, where it is required to block the channel. Recall that blocking the calcium channel is vital to preventing the influx of calcium into the cell, where it leads to the cell's destruction.

ANTIOXIDANTS

In the course of ordinary bodily functions and during ongoing metabolism, there are thousands of active chemical and biochemical reactions happening twenty-four hours a day, seven days a week in the human body. Some of the normal byproducts of these processes include waste products such as heat and, inevitably, oxidative stress.

Many of these waste products are unstable atoms and molecules known collectively as *free radicals*. Free radicals can directly damage any tissue, such as proteins and DNA. The creation of free radicals in the body is a natural occurrence and is accelerated by aging, as the body's levels of its naturally occurring antioxidants, such as hormones, decline.

Whenever there is tissue damage from an injury, especially of the ischemic type (which commonly happens in TBI), more than the usual amount of oxidative stress is created, which damages the tissues even further and leads to dysfunction.

An excellent example of cumulative oxidative stress is the consequence of the disease called aging. I call aging a disease because it fits the definition: a disease is any process that damages the body, whether by chemical, physical, or metabolic means. Just look at the average senior citizen, who appears frail, weak, and is typically taking a list of medications that may be causing secondary medical conditions as side effects, such as diabetes, ulcers, or hypertension from chronic steroid administration.

For these reasons we hear a lot about antioxidants, how good they are for our health, how they may help to reduce or prevent the impact of disease, and how they may lessen side effects from medications.

Effective plant-based antioxidants

Most people know that taking antioxidants is good for their health and that vitamins C and E are good sources of antioxidants, but what about others?

Many fruits and vegetables are concentrated sources of antioxidants, as antioxidants play a major role in preserving plant-based foods. Table 1 lists ten foods that are very high in antioxidants, with the highest source at the top and decreasing down the list.

Table 1. Top 10 High Antioxidant Foods

Food
Freeze-dried acai berries
Dark chocolate
Pecans
Elderberries
Wild blueberries

Artichoke (boiled)
Cranberries
Kidney beans
Blackberries
Goji berries

Antioxidant supplements

Supplements can be excellent sources of antioxidants when they are sourced from high-quality foods. The list of supplements that have a potent antioxidant effect is rather long, so only the most important and well-studied ones are described here.

Blueberries and pomegranates are at the top of the list of excellent antioxidant foods that are available in supplemental pill and liquid form. The antioxidant pycnogenol, or pine bark extract, helps with circulation by protecting the inner membrane of the arteries, supporting the healing of TBI.

Glutathione is one of the most important antioxidants in the body and especially the liver. Vitamin C plays a critical role in the function of glutathione, as the vitamin keeps the glutathione in a state that acts as an antioxidant. A precursor to glutathione is N-acetyl-cysteine (sold as the drug Mucomyst), which I often recommend to patients with liver problems, including hepatitis.

Resveratrol deserves special mention. This powerful antioxidant compound is found in red grapes, blueberries, cranberries, and dark chocolate, to name a few foods, and is readily available in supplement form. It is sometimes considered the "longevity" supplement because research has shown that it has a similar positive effect on the DNA as calorie restriction does. The science behind how resveratrol works indicates that the molecule penetrates the cell, enters the nucleus, and then connects to that portion of the DNA involved with turning on the genes of longevity.[3]

---

[3] These health benefits and others have been well described in a book called *The French Paradox and Beyond* by Lewis Perdue.

Lipoic acid is a well-known anti-inflammatory. It is one of the few supplements that is both water soluble and liposoluble, or soluble in both water and fat. (Recall that only liposoluble substances may enter the brain by passing through the BBB.) Once inside the brain, lipoic acid can perform the functions of both water and fat, which is advantageous. Lipoic acid is also a potent agent for enhancing mitochondrial function.

A final mention is a single product that contains many supplements that have individual health benefits as antioxidants. This proprietary product, called Cognitex®, is made by Life Extension and is designed to support cognitive function. It comes in several different forms.

High-quality supplements are an excellent approach to supporting the healing of brain injuries from TBI. When combined with other therapies, supplements can enhance and even accelerate the healing. When choosing supplements for whatever reason, always choose the highest quality possible, and remember to ask for laboratory proof of quality.

Chapter 12

Bio-Identical Hormone Therapy

Hormones regulate most of the body's vital functions ranging from energy levels to reproductive function, including many that act on a subconscious level. High or normal levels of hormones are associated with youth and vigor, whereas low levels correspond to old age, frailty, and disease states, including cancer.

Many symptoms may arise in those who have suffered a TBI, and some of them are related to hormonal imbalances. These imbalances, or more accurately, deficiencies, are related to injury to that part of the brain responsible for producing and transporting hormone-releasing factors to other parts of the body to their respective target organs.

THE PITUITARY GLAND

The pituitary gland (see fig. 11), sometimes called the master gland because it controls many hormones throughout the body, is located at the base of the brain inside a specialized bony structure called the *sella turcica* (Latin for "Turkish saddle"), so named because its shape resembles that of a saddle.

In humans, the gland is about the size of a pea. It has three distinct parts: the front part called the anterior or *adenohypophysis*; the middle section called the *intermediate lobe*; and the rear part called the *neurohypophysis*, the latter of which is connected to the hypothalamus by a thin, delicate structure called the *pituitary stalk*. This latter structure functions as a relay between the pituitary and the hypothalamus.

THE PITUITARY (HYPOPHYSIS) GLAND

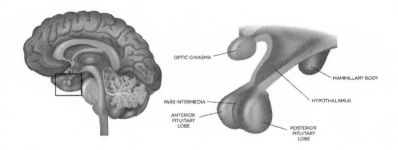

Figure 11. The pituitary gland.

The front, or anterior, portion of the pituitary gland is involved in the secretion of various hormones produced by at least five distinct, specialized secretory cells. The rear, or posterior, part of the pituitary, which is an extension of the hypothalamus, is connected via the stalk. It mainly receives hormones secreted by cells, and itself secretes two hormones: antidiuretic hormone and oxcytocin. The intermediate lobe, the smaller, third portion, plays a minor role in humans by producing *melanocyte-stimulating hormone*, which can also be secreted from the anterior portion.

Thus, the two main parts of the pituitary gland are the anterior and posterior lobes, each with quite different neuroanatomical descriptions. They both derive from distinct embryological origin and secrete distinct hormones.

The relationship between the hypothalamus and pituitary

The hypothalamus is located just above the pituitary gland at the base of the brain, just behind the frontal lobes and frontal bones. There is a special functional relationship between the hypothalamus, the pituitary gland, and target organs in the body. The sequence of functioning is as follows: The hypothalamus sends signals to the anterior pituitary gland via releasing factors for each respective hormone. Each releasing factor is named for the corresponding target cell in the pituitary gland. When the corresponding cell in the pituitary is stimulated, it responds by producing another hormone (one of seven), which is first secreted into the local circulation and then into the general (systemic) circulation.

This same hormone travels to its target organ, such as the ovaries, testicles, or kidneys. When the hormone reaches its specific receptor in the cell membrane, it stimulates the cell to produce its characteristic hormone, such as estrogen, progesterone, or testosterone.

This complex relationship, called the hypothalamic-pituitary axis, is under negative feedback control, meaning that when the hypothalamus detects low levels of hormones passing through the blood, it sends out a signal to release more releasing factors to increase that same hormone. The contrary is also true, such that a steady-state level of any hormone is maintained within a therapeutic range. The only exception to this rule is for oxytocin, secreted by the posterior pituitary gland, which is under control by a positive feedback loop system.

In such a delicate system, it is easy to imagine how damage to any part of the axis could disrupt the sequence of events needed to maintain hormonal stability, or homeostasis. In the case of trauma, several pathophysiological mechanisms have been identified, including direct damage to the area. Recall that the maximal force applied to the brain is in the frontal area, and that the inside surface of the skull is highly irregular, so it should not be surprising that direct damage may result when the bottom of the brain, where the hypothalamus is located, brushes up against the ragged inner surface of the skull. A common consequence of this trauma, seen in up to 43 percent of cases, is infarction (dead tissue) of the anterior pituitary gland.

Another mechanism for damage to the pituitary is inflammation in the area secondary to the trauma, which may compress the local tissues, much like when carpal tunnel syndrome develops in pregnant women as a result of fluid overload that compresses the median nerve in the tunnel of the wrist. Other mechanisms include bleeding with mass effect (and inflammatory edema) and fracture of the skull. Less frequently, stretching and/or tearing of the pituitary stalk can happen, causing either a partial or complete separation between the hypothalamus and the pituitary, which then causes the signaling between the two to be interrupted.

It is quite rare for me to hear any of my patients with mTBI complain of symptoms related to a loss of hormones as a result of hypopituitarism (low hormone production). Symptoms of hypopituitarism are primarily seen in moderate to severe TBIs and is not the focus in this discussion. Nevertheless, it is importance to recognize these types of symptoms and perform the appropriate laboratory testing. If low levels of hormones are confirmed, each deficiency should be treated with hormone replacement therapy.[4]

BIO-IDENTICAL HORMONE REPLACEMENT

When replacement hormones are prescribed, the most important factor is that they should only be of the type called *bio-identical*. This class of medication is made only in specialized compounding pharmacies.

It is important to know that bio-identical hormones are customized for specific deficiencies and should not be taken without a physician's supervision. The first step for patients with mTBI who think they may have hormone deficiencies is to have a blood panel performed to determine current levels of hormone production. Only then can the correct dosage be prescribed.

Bio-identical hormones have the identical molecular structure and function as the original hormone they are meant to replace, so the body recognizes the hormone as its own, and if dosed correctly,

---

[4] The interested reader is referred to the following articles: https://www.lifeextension.com/Magazine/2015/2/Heal-Traumatic-Brain-Injury-With-Bioidentical-Hormones/Page-01, and https://www.lifeextension.com/Magazine/2012/1/Using-Hormones-Heal-Traumatic-Brain-Injuries/Page-02.

there should be no side effects. The dosage has to be calculated based on the individual patient's needs, and no one dose fits all. The prescribing physician is therefore able to prescribe for specific concentrations of the medication instead of having to choose from what pharmaceutical companies make available.

Bio-identical HRT and pharmaceutical companies

Bio-identical hormones are not patentable, and thus there are few modern clinical trials on them, as pharmaceutical companies have no interest in paying for trials. In fact, pharmaceutical companies are in competition with bio-identical HRT, but their only products are synthetic hormones, which can cause many side effects.

Dosing forms of bio-identical hormones

The dosing forms for bio-identical hormones differ from standard pills. Formulations of bio-identical HRT come in creams, gels, and sublingual troches (lozenges), all designed to bypass the gastrointestinal system to prevent the medication from going to the liver, where it would be modified or metabolized into another molecule (called first-pass metabolism).

Hormones taken in pill form must pass through the liver, which alters their shape and function such that it becomes a different molecule, which means they will not have the exact function as the original and may even have other functions best described as side effects. In order to achieve the exact functions of the original molecule, its structure must not be altered.

The topical dosing forms, which include creams and gels, are applied to the skin, where they pass through and enter the bloodstream. It is important to apply topical drugs to areas of the body with the least amount of fat, as fat will absorb the hormone and reduce its bio-availability.

While topical medications can be applied in several places, I instruct my patients to apply the medication to the genital area to mimic where nature and biology have already determined as the best location and where evolution has proven effective.

Damage to the pituitary and hypothalamus glands can have devastating effects on hormone production and thus functions in the body regulated by hormones. Physician-prescribed bio-identical hormone replacement therapy usually helps by supplementing the body's low production of these hormones.

Chapter 13

Recovering from a TBI: Case Studies

I understand how frightening it is for a person to have suffered from a traumatic brain injury, which is why I feel it is so important to relate successful real-life cases that I have been directly involved with as the treating physician. My rational behind this approach is that if the treatment was successful for them, then it can be for you, your loved one, or anyone else you may know who suffers from TBI.

The first two cases I relate here were severe TBIs. Their stories will demonstrate that my treatment is effective and reverses all the aftereffects of a concussion, proven by scientific objective testing after treatment, with obvious improvement observed. If a treatment is successful in worst-case scenarios, then I believe it can be even more successful in milder cases.

CASE STUDY 1: JESSE V.

Jesse V., a healthy thirty-year-old male, came in to see me in August 1996 for an injury he had sustained in February 1995, about a year and a half earlier, which meant that he was not going to experience any further neurological recovery on his own, especially since he was undergoing aggressive multidisciplinary treatment. Jesse was referred to me his neuropsychologist, who was directing his rehabilitation.

Jesse's mother reported his history to me because Jesse had severe slurred speech and could not speak very well. His mother told me that he had been working as police officer in Hollywood, Florida. He was standing next to a car, apparently engaged in enforcing the law, when he was suddenly struck by another car, which catapulted him into the air such that he landed head first through the windshield, breaking numerous bones in his face, cheeks, and collar bone. He immediately lost consciousness and entered into a deep coma.

Jesse was admitted to the local hospital, which, lucky for him, was a level 1 trauma center. He was seen by a neurosurgeon for bleeding in the brain, who thought he was not a candidate for surgically evacuating the blood. The neurosurgeon told his mother that Jesse may not make it through the night.

But he did. Jesse remained in the ICU for three months, undergoing surgery to his face and for other numerous complications. He was then transferred to a rehabilitation facility, where he remained for six months, experiencing some degree of recovery. He was then transferred to a nursing home, where he stayed for eight months. He finally went home under the care of his mother.

Jesse was referred to me to specifically address his symptoms of violent and aggressive behavior, both provoked and spontaneous. Other symptoms included severe slurred speech, poor short-term memory, drooling, depression, anger, and motor impairment, with weakness in the right side of his body greater than the left side. He was not able to walk and was confined to a wheelchair.

Jesse's medical history was unremarkable, and he had not had any previous head trauma. He was taking numerous medications, including strong antipsychotic drugs such as Haldol, to control his outbursts, but they were not working well. His neurological examination revealed a markedly impaired individual who required assistance to transfer from his wheelchair onto the examination table. I found that he had evidence of previous facial surgery, a tracheostomy scar, generalized muscular atrophy worse on the right than left, and a dependent redness of the lower extremities, all as a result of the accident.

The cranial nerve examination showed that Jesse had facial weakness in the lower part of his face, with the right side weaker than the left. The motor examination showed he had muscle contraction (spasticity) that was worse on the right than the left, except at the ankles. He had marked weakness (pronator drift) in the arms, worse on the right than the left, although his strength was excellent in the shoulders, with only slight weakness on the right greater than left.

His grip was stronger in his left hand, but rapid alternating movements were markedly impaired, again worse on the right than left. (Rapid alternating movements are movements such as quickly tapping the index finger to the thumb up and down.) Jesse's legs demonstrated more weakness than his arms. He had a foot drop in both feet and was unable to bend his feet downward. His knees were moderately weak, more so on the right than the left.

Jesse's reflexes were abnormal, too brisk and asymmetric, and brisker on the right than the left. The reflex on the sole of his right foot was neutral, whereas a normal response is that the toes move downward. The same reflex on his left foot was clearly normal.

A cerebellar examination reviews a patient's conscious regulation of balance, muscle tone, and coordination of voluntary movements. I could perform Jesse's cerebellar exam only by observation because he was unable to cooperate. It showed that he had marked instability when he was sitting, as he would fall to the right. He was unable to perform routine tests of coordination because he was so impaired, and as mentioned, he could not walk at all.

Simple tests of Jesse's sensations were difficult to interpret, although there didn't appear to be any asymmetry to pinprick or temperature. More complicated sensory testing requires a normal functioning cortex. For example, one test called graphesthesia of the palms is where a number is drawn in the palm of the patient's hand, and the patient is asked to report what the number is. Jesse was unable to perceive any numbers I drew with my finger in either of his hands.

My initial diagnostic impression was traumatic brain injury of the severe type, along with residual post-concussion syndrome, loss of speech, slurred speech, and left greater than right hemispheric dysfunction. Behavioral problems, including both provoked and unprovoked aggressive behavior, ruled out partial complex seizure disorder, which is seizure that starts in one area of the brain and causes the person to have altered consciousness and abnormal behavioral patterns.

I ordered Jesse to have EEG, QEEG, and QEP; SPECT of the brain; and MRI of the brain. I also ordered his medical records from the hospital where he was seen initially and from the rehabilitation center.

Jesse had a significantly abnormal MRI of the brain. There was evidence for extensive cortical and subcortical tissue loss (infarction) in the frontal and temporal cortices. The location of this infarct (a localized area of tissue loss) was consistent with head trauma. He also had associated volume loss in all parts of his brain, indicating shrinkage, called *atrophy*. I noted a small area of white matter signal abnormality in the right frontal and parietal region, which may have been due to a shear injury (diffuse axonal injury, as described in chapter 1). The interpretation of this report means that Jesse had generalized shrinkage of the brain, both in both hemispheres and in the brainstem, indicating a severe brain injury, particularly because the brain stem was affected.

I performed and interpreted Jesse's EEG testing, QEEG test, and a battery of QEPs. He was difficult to test because he was agitated and uncooperative and had to be sedated with Valium, which calmed him down but also changed his background electrical activity by increasing the fast brain waves (beta waves).

My impression of the standard EEG was that it was within normal limits. However, his QEEG and QEP were significantly abnormal. (This is an example of the difference between EEG and QEEG.) I reviewed all of the various focal abnormalities and found that there were sixty-two focal abnormalities in the left hemisphere and thirty-two in the right. My overall impression was that Jesse's brain was moderately abnormal on the left and mildly abnormal on the right.

In a follow-up visit with Jesse and his mother, I decided to videotape him in order to make a record of his pre-treatment status.

After the videotaping, we planned for Jesse to start treatment with nimodipine to increase blood flow to his brain, and hyperbaric oxygen therapy (HBOT) to increase the oxygen in his blood. You can see the videotape of Jesse's pre-treatment status by following the link in the footnote.[5]

Jesse had a brainstem auditory evoked response (BAER) performed to assess for dizziness. This test has two parts, one to test the brainstem and the other to test the cortex (see BAER in chapter 7). Both parts were abnormal, providing objective evidence that there was 1) a loss of power, mostly on the left side of the brain, and 2) damage to both the brainstem (left and right) and the cortex, as the signal from the brainstem to the cortex was delayed.

He also had a Ceretec SPECT scan, which showed the expected findings of hypoperfusion (low blood flow) in the usual front-to-back gradient (as described in chapter 1). But the scan was markedly abnormal because there was no blood flow in the left frontotemporal parietal lobes (the area of prior bleeding), indicating that there was dead tissue there and in the basal ganglia. I also detected areas of hypoperfusion in the left and right frontal lobes. There were lesser degrees of hypoperfusion in the rear of the left hemisphere, including the occipital lobe, and scattered portions of the right frontal and parietal lobes.

Figure 12 shows 3-D reconstructed computerized images from Jesse's SPECT scan. The top left upper image (image 1) is the anterior view (looking straight on), and image 9 (counting left to right, top to bottom) is the posterior view (looking from the back of the brain). The rest of the top row shows views of the right side of the brain, and the bottom row shows views of the left side. Note the multiple defects seen as black holes, and that they are worse on the left side compared to the right.

---

[5] To view a pre-post video of Jesse's post-treatment status, see https://youtu.be/f1JQL4ssFD8. In the pre-treatment video Jesse is wearing a plaid shirt and in the post-treatment video he is wearing a black vest over a shirt.

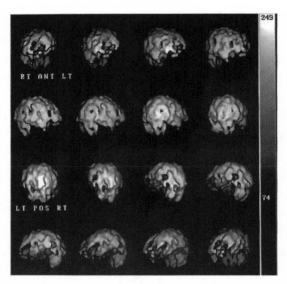

Figure 12. A SPECT scan of patient Jesse's brain before treatment. These reconstructed 3-D computerized images show the hypoperfusion in the cortex.

Jesse came in for a follow-up visit about three months later. Since his last visit, he had been taking nimodipine 30 mg three times a day and going to HBOT on a daily basis. I noted that he had increased alertness and awareness but his outbursts had increased, although he was not physically abusing anyone as before. Also, immediately after leaving the HBOT chamber after each treatment, his speech became significantly clearer and therefore easier to understand. I thought he was beginning to respond to the treatment and recommended that his nimodipine be gradually increased.

In December 1996 he had another follow-up visit. He had continued to go to HBOT every day for an hour at a time. I increased his nimodipine, and he was able to tolerate two capsules of 30 mg three times a day, for total of 180 mg a day. Everybody involved with his care had noted a distinct improvement in his condition, most notably because his speech had become clearer and was now understandable.

Jesse's aggressive behavior had decreased significantly, to the point where he no longer needed antipsychotic medications, and his sedatives were decreased. A neurological examination showed an increased strength of his right side, and his left side was essentially at full power. He did have moderate weakness of the right hand, and his rapid alternating movements were still significantly decreased, again right greater than left, although he was able to attempt rapid alternating movement with his right hand. Significantly, he was able to perform and cooperate when I examined him, which he could not do before.

At this point, I recommended that Jesse increase the nimodipine again, to three capsules three times a day, and complete forty-five more hyperbaric treatments (I had ordered ninety). I also recommended that he be re-scanned with SPECT and repeat the quantitative EEG and quantitative EPs after he completed the full ninety treatments of HBOT.

In late January 1997, Jesse had another Ceretec SPECT scan, which was done at the same facility so that a valid comparison could be made between the pre-and post-treatment scans (this is important for all comparative scans.) The comparative impression showed that Jesse had experienced significant improvement, as seen in the post-treatment SPECT scan. There was evidence of normalized perfusion in the entire right hemisphere, and a significant improvement of perfusion in all parts of the left hemisphere except for the area of residual decreased or absent blood flow in the lower part of the left frontal lobe and portions of the junction of the temporal and parietal lobes.

Of note, this second SPECT was performed after sixty-two HBOT treatments. Jesse had improved so much that I sent him for the second scan early instead of waiting until after ninety HBOT sessions, as originally planned. Following the second SPECT scan, he did complete the full ninety treatments of HBOT.

Figure 13b shows Jesse's post-treatment 3-D SPECT, in which can be seen the cortical perfusion (blood flow in the cortex). The areas of white are normal, indicating adequate perfusion of the brain. The dark areas represent places where there is still decreased blood flow, and the parts of the brain that are missing on the left side (ragged, irregular surfaces) are areas of dead or lost brain tissue. For comparison, the pre-treatment scan is shown again in figure 13a.

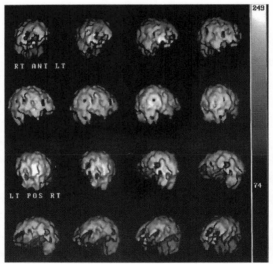

Figure 13a: The SPECT scan of Jesse's brain before treatment.

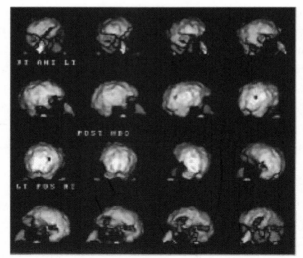

Figure 13b. The SPECT scan of Jesse's brain after treatment.

The top row in figure 13a shows the front of the brain, and the bottom row shows the left side of the brain, where the bleeding and maximal injury occurred. Note that the entire right side of the brain is white and smooth, indicating normal blood flow except for a tiny area in the back on the right side (third row, first image).

Note that in the left side of the brain in figure 13b, many areas appear white and thus normal, whereas other areas still appear dark and irregular, indicating low or no blood flow as a result of the tissue loss from the severe injury and bleeding. The left side still has more and larger perfusion defects, which are seen as black holes, than on the right side, although we can still see improvement compared to the pre-treatment scan. Note the right side appears more white or normal except for a tiny spot in the right occipital lobe.

Jesse improved considerably from all points of view, and I videotaped him again to document his clinical improvement. The video shows that he presented as a very different person compared to when I first saw him, and he was cooperative and calm in demeanor. He was able to comprehend most verbal commands and follow complex commands. In fact, some aspects of the examination that he could not do at all before treatment he was now able to do, which also represented an improvement.

Jesse's motor strength improved to normal except for his right hand, which was only mildly weak. He did have significant slowing of the rapid alternating movements, right greater than left, but the prior weakness in both feet was completely resolved. His reflexes remained pathological, increased on the right, and the plantar response was normal on the left and still abnormal on the right. To see a video of Jesse's improvement, follow the link in the footnote.[6]

CASE STUDY 2: SYLVIE W.

Sylvie W. was a thirty-year-old woman who was referred to me by Gerald Gluck, PhD, a neurofeedback therapist and colleague who

---

[6] To view video of Jesse's pre and post-treatment see https://youtu.be/f1JQL4ssFD8. In the pre-treatment video Jesse is wearing a plaid shirt and in the post-treatment video he is wearing a black vest over a shirt.

performed Sylvie's QEEG. I first saw Sylvie in January 2015, eight years and eight months after her injury in an accident in May 2006.

Sylvie was a passenger in the front seat of a car and was wearing her seatbelt. A rapidly moving Dodge Durango truck struck the passenger side of the vehicle and literally crushed it. The impact was so violent that the car Sylvie was in was knocked into two poles and flew into three other cars. When the paramedics arrived at the scene, they thought she was already dead, but then they heard faint breathing sounds. Further assessment by the paramedics revealed that her Glasgow Coma Scale was 3-15 (3 out of 15; the scale is 3 [deep coma] to 15 [fully awake]), indicating that she was in a coma and that she had sustained a severe TBI. Rescuers used the "jaws of life" for forty-five minutes to extract her from the vehicle. The doctors in the emergency room thought that she would not survive, but she surprised everyone.

Sylvie's initial MRI brain scan was performed four days after her injury. It showed severe and multiple hemorrhagic contusions in the right greater than left frontal lobes, the right temporal lobe, the left thalamus, and the left side of the brainstem. There was also blood in the ventricles. Recall the gradient of injury discussed previously, when the force applied to the brain begins in the front and propagates from superficial to deep. Injury to deep structures such as the brainstem, which Sylvie sustained, are objective evidence of a severe injury.

After two weeks in the ICU, Sylvie opened her eyes, but she was completely non-responsive. She was transferred to a trauma unit for six weeks, and was discharged home almost two months after the accident. She required total at-home care around the clock. She did begin to make some sort of recovery but only very gradually, and over many months.

Sylvie had never had comprehensive aggressive treatment, but she did have some official treatment (three to four hours a day for five weeks) when she was seen at a facility in Phoenix, Arizona, in October 2014.

She had a CT brain scan performed in November 2014, many years after the injury and about six weeks before coming to South Florida. The report from the scan indicated that she had mild swelling in the right frontal scalp, where the impact to her brain occurred. There was interval resolution, or improvement, of the hemorrhages and dead brain tissue in the right frontotemporal lobes, was unchanged from a prior study in June 2010. Although the report did not mention any cerebral atrophy (shrinkage), it is almost certain that it was present.

Another MRI of Sylvie's brain was performed in July 2015 and compared to the study from 2006. The areas of the dead brain tissue in the right frontotemporal lobes were unchanged, although the study described for the first time that there was mild to moderate cerebral and cerebellar atrophy, but no mention of brainstem atrophy.

When Sylvie first came to my office, she couldn't walk and was in a wheelchair. Her head was tilted to her left because she had lost part of her visual field on the left, and by tilting her head, she was able to see out of the remaining portion of her right visual field. She wore a special brace on her right lower leg and foot. She was unable to speak but appeared to understand simple commands.

Sylvie's SPECT scan was performed in January 2015 on a triple-head, state-of-the-art instrument with statistical analysis. The numerous abnormalities seen in the scan matched the findings on her prior MRI and CT scans. Images of slices of the brain showed there was severe hypoperfusion in the right frontal areas in two specific areas that corresponded to two different arteries. The latter is seen even better in the 3-D views, which show a clear delineation of the two separate areas of decreased blood flow (figs. 14 and 15).

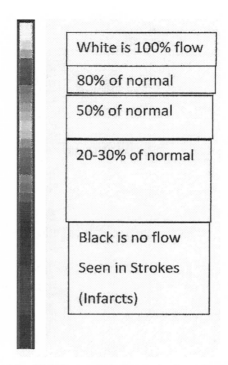

Figure 14. Legend for SPECT scans. This flow scale shows how to interpret the next figure.

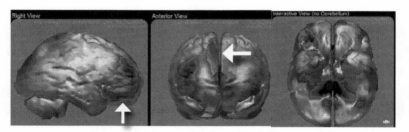

Figure 15. A computerized 3-D image of Sylvie's SPECT scan. The scan on the left shows the right side of the brain; the center is taken from the front, looking head-on, and the right is a bottom view looking up, with the front of the brain at the top.

The dark color in figure 15 indicates a severe loss of blood flow to those areas of the brain. Note the severe hypoperfusion seen in dark shades and black in the right frontal lobe (*left*), the right temporal lobe (*center*), and the rear ventral junction with the front ventral occipital lobe.

Sylvie's EEG report was definitely abnormal, as confirmed by the numerous visible abnormalities. Most of them were on the right side of the brain, although the left temporal lobe was worse than the right. Some of the findings were related to cortical irritability (seizure-like activity in the brain), which can also be seen in epilepsy. The findings of right abnormalities greater than left, combined with a history of trauma from the right side, is suggestive of a coup contrecoup-type injury.

Standard deviation

A statistical analysis compares the individual to a group norm. A difference between the individual in question and the group norm is described as a deviation. The deviation can be quantified by either a plus (+) or a minus (−) sign, denoting too much or too little compared to the norm. This type of analysis is objective and more scientific than someone's opinion about whether or not something is normal.

Sylvie's scans demonstrate that the hypoperfusion corresponds to a negative deviation at −2 to greater than −4, with maximal loss of perfusion in the front compared to the back gradient (see figure 16). The white arrows in figure 16 point to the areas of maximum deviation, which is greater than −4.

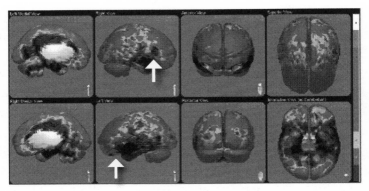

Figure 16. 3-D computerized statistical analyses in the right/left sides and anterior views and bottom views, showing maximum deviation.

I videotaped Sylvie to preserve her pre-treatment neurological status. (Follow the link in the footnote to view the video.[7]) Since she was from out of town, we agreed that she would undergo an extremely intensive treatment. After her initial diagnostic workup, she went for neurofeedback twice a day and HBOT treatment once a day. I saw her on a weekly basis to monitor her condition and to escalate her dose of nimodipine, which I did on an almost weekly basis for a total of six weeks.

As with Jesse V., Sylvie's neurological symptoms significantly decreased after treatment. Some of her vision returned, which enabled her to sit with her head upright since she could now see out of most of her visual field. Her gag reflex returned, which permitted her to eat without the risk of choking (which may result in aspiration pneumonia).

I reevaluated Sylvie between the fifth and sixth weeks after her treatment because she had to return to Canada. Again, there appeared to be a dramatic difference in her performance in that now she was able to get up onto the examination table, albeit with assistance; she was holding her head up straight, and she no longer needed the brace on her right foot. The stiffness of her legs because of spasticity still did not allow her legs to bend fully at the knees,

---

[7] To view a video of Sylvie's pre-treatment see https://youtu.be/-_fGMpDysxc

but she could sit on the exam table with her legs held out straight, the right more than the left. She also regained some strength of her right side. Her left side did not demonstrate any weakness at all.

Sylvie was able to verbalize some words although her voice was very weak. She was cognitively more intact, and overall, there was significant improvement in her neurological status. I believe that everyone was pleased with her progress, which was achieved in just six weeks. (To view Sylvie's post-treatment video, click on the link in the footnote.[8])

The fact that Sylvie, who was injured more severely than Jesse V., and the fact that she showed so much neurological recovery in only six weeks almost nine years after her injury, is indeed quite remarkable and encouraging. Had she been able to stay longer to continue her intensive treatment, she would have made an even a greater recovery.

Some time after Sylvie returned home, she sent me an email with a video of her at home. In the video, she ascends a winding staircase, with a little assistance, in her bare feet. At the time that I was treating her, she would not have been able to perform this activity. Clearly, she has continued to make further neurological recovery many years after the original injury, which never occurs spontaneously. In other words, the treatment was effective. The link to that video is in the footnote.[9]

CASE STUDY 3: MICHAEL W.

The third case, that of twenty-two-year-old Michael W., differs from the first two cases in that it represents what is called a typical mTBI, even though the impact on Michael's life could not have been considered mild, since it interrupted his entire life as a college student.

Prior to seeing me in February 2017, Michael had seen Dr. Gluck, who had performed a QEEG that was significantly abnormal. He

[8] To view a video of Sylvie's post-treatment see https://youtu.be/NPIp0A9WC-I
[9] To view a video of Sylvie walking up a flight of stairs, please see https://youtu.be/XheRL-2i4NvA

had been undergoing neurofeedback and was referred to me for neurological evaluation because of a deterioration in his ability to perform well at school.

Michael was a personable and bright young man who had generally done well academically, as seen in his acceptance at a top-tier undergraduate school. He had also excelled in sports, including in varsity in college. He had been playing soccer, including doing headers, since he was young. He had continued doing these moves until shortly before I saw him. Michael denied that he had had loss of consciousness (LOC) or concussions from any of these actions but admitted to numerous incidents of "having his bell rung" and then shaking off the change of awareness. He had likely suffered numerous minor head injuries related to sports.

Suddenly, in the prior couple of semesters, Michael, who normally got A's and B's, suffered problems with learning, executive functions, and memory, resulting in failing grades. Based on interview and test results, I determined that this decline was caused by cumulative mTBIs. Symptoms of such injuries may take as long as ten years to manifest, and may therefore catch the patient by surprise.

Michael's QEEG was abnormal, especially in the left frontal lobe, and the right more so than the left temporal, parietal, and occipital lobes. The findings were consistent with the trauma he disclosed in his history of playing soccer for many years and one year of playing American football.

His neurological exam was mostly normal except for a minor impairment of balance when he stood on one foot with his eyes closed, and it was worse on the left than the right. With his history and mostly normal neurological examination, one would never think he had a serious neurological condition. The initial diagnostic impression was history of academic deterioration, history of remote and repetitive trauma, and history of abnormal QEEG. I still needed to rule out hypoperfusion. Michael was sent for a SPECT of the brain. To my surprise, his study was significantly abnormal.

Two-dimensional slices of his brain indicated areas of decreased blood flow, and 3-D images of the raw data showed a decrease of perfusion in a pattern characteristic of trauma. Other 3-D images showed multiple defects, which are clearly seen as dark areas and depressions (see fig. 17). These can also be seen at the bottom of the raw data, which confirms the hypoperfusion characteristic of trauma.

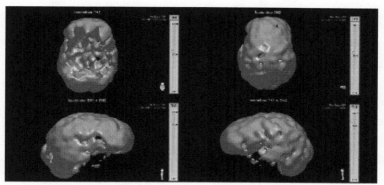

Figure 17. 3-D reconstructed images showing multiple defects.

Figure 18 represents a statistical analysis of Michael's perfusion compared to a normative database that is stored in the program. The widespread hypoperfusion is statistically quite significant and corresponds to varying degrees of hypoperfusion. The areas of maximal hypoperfusion are denoted by the black colors.

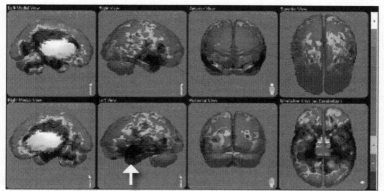

Figure 18. A pre-treatment 3-D SPECT scan showing the statistical analysis. Black areas represent maximum deviation (maximum abnormal).

The overall impression of Michael's SPECT scan was that it was abnormal because of hypoperfusion in the left greater than right temporal lobes and right greater than left frontal lobes. Overall, Michael's SPECT was a moderately to severely abnormal study. The gradient of damage, from the front toward the rear, and left greater than right, was consistent with a history of trauma and concussions. The distribution of the hypoperfusion seen on his pre-treatment SPECT scan matches that of the QEEG, which was performed prior to the SPECT. It establishes the abnormalities and reinforces the accuracy of the findings.

Much to my surprise, not only was Michael's scan abnormal, it was severely abnormal in certain lobes such as the temporal lobes, and it was asymmetric, worse on the left than right. Moreover, the pattern was typical for a coup contrecoup trauma. The lesson I learned in this case was that even a detailed clinical neurological examination is not sensitive enough to confirm a diagnosis of post-concussion syndrome, and that SPECT and QEEG are much more sensitive tests at picking up objective abnormalities.

I gave Michael a prescription for nimodipine 30 mg four times a day and suggested that he continue the neurofeedback with Dr. Gluck.

Second SPECT scan

Michael had a follow-up visit in May 2017. He had added HBOT to his treatment protocol by then and had had about twenty-seven treatments. He reported significant improvement, especially in his cognitive skills, including his memory.

He had a second SPECT scan performed that month, which showed significant increase of blood flow in several areas of the brain, but the left anterior pole of the left temporal lobe, which was his worse area, was still very hypoperfused, thus indicating that he needed more treatment. I increased his dosage of nimodipine to two caps four times a day.

The second scan was still abnormal, with widespread moderate to severe hypoperfusion in the left greater than right temporal lobe, and more so than the frontal lobes. However, areas that had been less severely abnormal had normalized, and areas of more severe hypoperfusion were less so. The second scan also showed a significant increase of perfusion, especially in the inferior frontal lobes (right greater than left), the central lobes, and the parietal lobes. His treatments were clearly making a difference.

Third SPECT scan

Michael had a third scan and another follow-up visit in July 2017. By this time, he was taking two caps of 30 mg nimodipine three times a day for a total of 180 mg per day, was receiving LORETA neurofeedback, and had completed forty-one HBOT.

I compared this most recent scan with his first one from February 2017. It showed a significant increase of perfusion, most prominently in the frontal lobes, especially in the right hemisphere; in the central lobe just superior to the temporal lobe; and in the parietal lobe. The previously severe hypoperfusion in the left temporal lobe was not significantly changed.

My impression of the third scan was that it was a persistently abnormal study, with evidence of both treatment effect and significant hypoperfusion, particularly in the left anterior temporal lobe. However, when compared with previous scans, in particular his pre-treatment study of February 2017, there was a significant increase of perfusion, especially in the right central lobe and the left frontal lobe. There was also a relative increase of perfusion in the bilateral frontal lobes.

Since the right hemisphere was not as severely affected as the left hemisphere, it was logical that the least affected part of the brain would respond faster than the more affected left hemisphere. The bottom surface of the brain remained severe, but the area affected was significantly less in size compared to the prior study.

Michael came in for a follow-up in August 2017 to review the SPECT performed the previous month. During that visit, he reported that he was still undergoing LORETA neurofeedback twice a week and had completed about seventy HBOT treatments.

Fourth SPECT scan

Michael came in for a fourth SPECT scan in September 2017. I could not see significant increased perfusion by visual inspection compared to the second study in May 2017, but a statistical analysis of the differences between the two scans did show relative increases in small, discrete areas in the frontal lobes, the left posterior frontal, and the left central lobe close to the junction with the temporal lobe (see fig. 19).

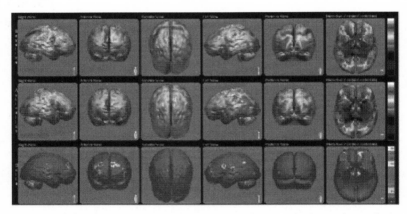

Figure 19. Michael's SPECT scan post-treatment. The top row shows the perfusion before treatment; the middle row shows the post-treatment perfusion, and the bottom row shows the difference between the two studies. The statistical difference and the colors in the bottom row show an increase of perfusion equal to 1.5 to 2.5 deviations from the norm.

The scan also showed that there was still severe hypoperfusion. The only apparent area of improvement was in the left frontal lobe, which showed a significant improvement. The scan was still abnormal, with evidence of severe hypoperfusion in the left greater than right temporal lobes, and in the temporal lobes into both occipital lobes. However, there was one area of improved perfusion in the left frontal lobe.

Standard deviation by color

For a statistical analysis of a patient's individual perfusion compared against a normative database with age match control, if the patient's perfusion is significantly less than normal, and it exceeds 2 standard deviations, then it is abnormal with a 95 percent degree of confidence, denoted by colder colors of teal to light blue and then dark blue. If the perfusion exceeds 3 deviations, the confidence level rises to 99.5 percent. On the other hand, a relative increase of perfusion corresponds to a positive deviation denoted by hot colors, starting with red, magenta, and white (to see the colors please refer to the digital version).

Note that on this fourth scan there is improvement in perfusion in the left front lobe for the first time, but there is still significant hypoperfusion in the left anterior temporal lobe, the area of prior maximum abnormality. Michael was instructed to continue with his treatment, complete his HBOT treatments, and return for follow-up evaluation.

CASE STUDY 4: JOHN W.

John W., a twenty-one-year-old male, was referred to me by Dr. Gluck, his neurofeedback therapist. He is also the brother of Michael W., the subject of case study 3. John was seen for depression with suicidal ideation, and later for loss of motivation that had caused him to deteriorate academically, from achieving A's in his classes to getting much poorer grades.

John had a significant medical history of two episodes of head trauma. The first one occurred at age four. He was playing soccer when he hit his head on a brick wall, sustaining a hematoma. He went to the emergency room for a medical evaluation, but it is unknown if he had a brain scan. The second episode happened at age fourteen. He was playing goalkeeper at a soccer game. He was hit in the head and knocked unconscious for one minute. He did not have any symptoms of a concussion, so a medical evaluation was not undertaken.

Following John's initial consultation, my diagnostic impression was history of depression, loss of motivation, and academic deterioration. A detailed neurological examination showed a small degree of left frontal lobe dysfunction, and probably right parietal lobe dysfunction, as well. The latter finding, coupled with a history of head trauma, was suggestive of a coup contrecoup-type injury. My initial recommendation was to review the recently performed QEEG, order a SPECT of John's brain, and send him for laboratory testing, including hormones.

In July 2016, John had the QEEG. I found that the QEEG analyses were deviant from normal and showed impairment in the right greater then left frontal lobes, in the left greater than right temporal lobes and parietal lobes, especially in the left parietal lobe. The LORETA test was abnormal in parts of the frontal lobes.

John's concussion index (see chapter 7, fig. 9) was abnormal and showed vulnerability in his distractibility, memory, mood, and executive function. *Coherence*, a measure of connectivity, showed decreased functional connectivity and efficiency, with patterns of long-paired increased coherence (too much connectivity at long distances, such as between the frontal and occipital lobes) and short-paired decreased coherence (too little connectivity within an individual lobe, such as the frontal lobe). This latter finding has been associated with mild trauma to the head.

Paradoxically, John presented with superior cognitive ability and felt satisfied with his overall functioning, except for incidents of depression. Nevertheless, the data indicated vulnerabilities. Though there was no evidence or appearance that he was involved in substance abuse, I recommended that it was best that he avoided drugs of abuse. Similarly, it was best if he avoided sports activities that involve contact and risk of head injury.

John had a Ceretec SPECT scan in August 2016. In the 3-D reconstructed images of the raw data, there was very clear hypoperfusion in the temporal lobes, confirming what was seen on the 2-D. There was also hypoperfusion seen in the right parietal lobe. In the back of the brain, both occipital lobes were under-perfused. In addition, there was significant hypoperfusion in the bottom of the bilateral frontal lobes, bilateral temporal lobes, and the front part of the occipital lobes. Both inferior frontal lobes were also significantly hypoperfused (see figs. 20a and 20b).

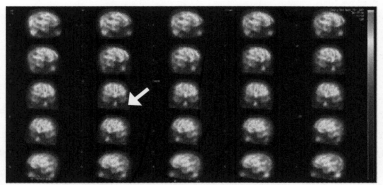

Figure 20a. Pre-treatment SPECT scan, front-of-the-brain view.

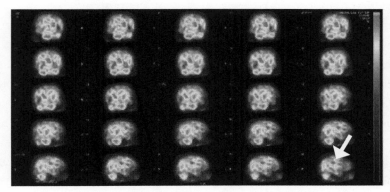

Figure 20b. Pre-treatment SPECT scan, rear and right-side views.

My overall impression was a moderate to severely abnormal Ceretec SPECT scan with evidence of hypoperfusion seen in the left greater than right temporal lobes, left slightly greater than right frontal lobes, left greater than right occipital lobes, and right significantly more than left parietal lobes hypoperfusion. The latter, coupled with John's history of trauma, is characteristic of a coup contrecoup-type injury.

In August 2016, John had a follow-up visit. I reviewed the SPECT of his brain with John and his father. On the basis of the hypoperfusion just described, I gave John a prescription for nimodipine 30 mg to be taken three times a day and a prescription for HBOT. He was getting neurofeedback during his short stay here in Florida, and I recommended that he find a neurofeedback therapist where he was going to college in Virginia.

John had another follow-up visit in February 2017. He reported that he was taking nimodipine 30 mg a day but was unable to get neurofeedback back at home in Texas. He did feel that the nimodipine helped him in terms of improved academic performance, improved duration of his ability to sit and study, and the resulting higher grades. I reviewed his laboratory data from July 2016. His testosterone was low, but his libido and performance weren't affected. His vitamin D3 was very low, but he had stopped taking the supplement because he lost the bottle. I recommended that he increase the nimodipine to four capsules a day.

John had his last follow-up in May 2017. Since his February visit, he had been taking nimodipine four times a day. He was also able to go back to HBOT and had had about twenty-two treatments at that point. He was off from college for that semester, but clinically, he felt he was improved, as demonstrated by his increased motivation to go back to school. He also had another post-treatment SPECT scan, which demonstrated a significant increase of perfusion.

In all of his 2-D imaging planes, the areas of hypoperfusion seen before were still present but to a lesser degree as a result of the treatment effect (see fig. 21).

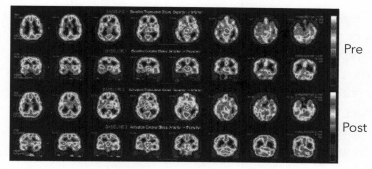

Figure 21. John's post-treatment SPECT scan. The top two rows of images are 2-D slices before treatment in the axial plane *(top row)* and coronal plane *(second row)*. The bottom two rows are the post-treatment scans in the same order. They show increased perfusion in multiple areas of the brain.

The post-treatment scans showed a relative increase of perfusion in areas previously under-perfused; in areas of maximal hypoperfusion, there was still significant hypoperfusion but less than on the pre-treatment images. The hypoperfusion was still asymmetric but had decreased more on the left, with maximum in the left greater than right temporal lobes. I also noted that there had been a considerable increase of perfusion of the left greater than right cerebellum.

The areas of increased perfusion are more clearly seen in 3-D reconstructed computerized images, especially in the left temporal lobe, the right central lobe, the left occipital lobe, and the left cerebellum (see fig. 22).

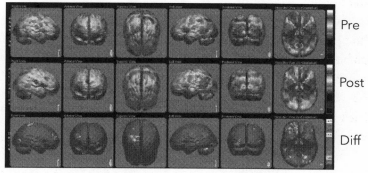

Figure 22. Pre and post-treatment scans (top and middle), and the differences between them *(bottom)*.

The top row of images in the figure is the baseline study of August 2016, the second row is the more recent study of May 2017, and the third row is the difference between the two, called the delta. The areas of maximum improvement are the right inferior frontal lobe, the right central lobe, and the left cerebellum, as seen in the third row. Compared to the pre-treatment scan, there was considerable improvement of perfusion.

In May 2017(seen in fig. 23, 24) I recommended that John increase the dose of nimodipine to two capsules three times a day for a total of 180 mg a day, continue the HBOT, and commence LORETA neurofeedback, since he was finally able to find a provider.

John had another SPECT scan performed in September 2017, seen in figures 23/24, which showed additional but lesser improvements compared to his last scan seen in figure 20a/b.

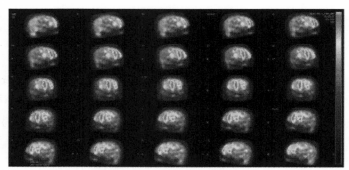

Figure 23. Final SPECT scan post-treatment, front-of-the-brain view.

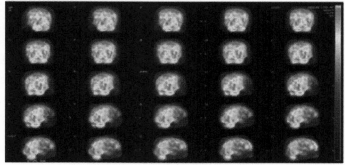

Figure 24. Final SPECT scan post-treatment, rear and side views.

A comparison of the 3-D computerized reconstructed images reveals small areas of increased perfusion in the front of both frontal lobes (underneath aspect), the rear part of the left frontal lobe, and the junction where the temporal lobes meet the central lobe.

Finally, figure 25 shows a comparative statistical analysis demonstrating a relative improvement in the left inferior frontal lobe.

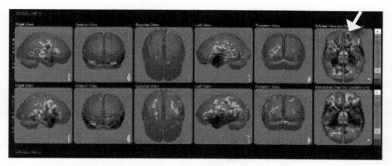

Figure 25. Post-treatment scan. The top row shows the statistical analysis during treatment. The bottom row shows the same but at the end of the treatment period. The main findings are noted in the left frontal lobe on the bottom surface.

My impression of the final scan was a persistently abnormal SPECT scan with severe hypoperfusion in the left greater than right temporal lobes, the bottom inner aspect of the temporal/occipital lobes, the left greater than right posterior temporal lobes, and to a lesser extent both frontal lobes (underneath aspect). John also had relative improvement of perfusion in the left inferior frontal lobe. Overall, this last scan was a persistently moderate-to-severe abnormal SPECT with mild improvement in the left inferior frontal lobe.

The improvement was significant in various parts of John's brain, especially the bottom of the left frontal lobe, even though there was still severe hypoperfusion in some places. It also told me that the treatment was partially successful and that he required more time in treatment to achieve an even better response. He noticed the improvements and attributed them to the treatments.

RECOVERY FROM A TBI

I have reported on four different cases of TBI with post-concussion symptoms in this chapter. Two of them were of the severe type, and two were what is classified as mild, or mTBI. In all cases, each patient experienced significant clinical improvement after treatment, as measured by both relative and absolute standards. The relative measure is the difference between the baseline (original) clinical state and subsequent states, whereas the absolute measure is the objective improvements compared to a normal population. These measures are disclosed by tests such as the SPECT and QEEG.

I have observed areas of hypoperfusion in the brain that were deviant from normal before treatment return to normal after treatment, and other areas with even greater hypoperfusion greatly improve. Depending on the individual, the relative difference between where they started and where they improved to can make the difference between succeeding in school and dropping out, or between going back to work and having to be on disability. These clinical observations, which I see on a regular basis in this particular population of patients, have permitted me to predict the outcome for patients utilizing my protocol as described.

I would like to leave this chapter with the following conclusion: if these four patients experienced significant healing of their brains from their injuries despite how severe they were or how many years had gone by, you or your loved one can, too. It does not matter how a person was concussed, or when, or how many times. The mechanism of injury is the same as has been described in detail, and the treatment is the same, although it may take longer for some than others.

Chapter 14

Long-Term Complications

Some TBI patients wonder if they are susceptible to long-term complications such as Alzheimer's disease or Parkinson's disease. The short answer is yes, but the long answer requires a more thorough explanation.

Recall from chapters 2 and 3 how the brain is damaged from the physical and biochemical cascades of events that lead to neuronal death. Recall as well that each neuron has 10 thousand connections, to other cells. The diversity of synaptic connections between millions of neurons within functional units known as hubs is what drives and maintains the brain's health and proper functioning.

Many neurons, and therefore synaptic connections, are lost when the brain is concussed. This loss contributes to a relative reduction in the proper functioning, and especially the connectivity, between neurons, which can be measured via QEEG tests. The overall effect is to lessen the brain's power output, reduce its speed and efficiency, and likely lower the IQ. This process is analogous to the metabolic insult to the brain caused by Alzheimer's, albeit via different mechanisms.

There is a long and diverse history of literature relating TBI to the development of Alzheimer's, yet there is also more recent research refuting the same, thereby raising the notion that TBI predisposing one to developing Alzheimer's is controversial. One review article concluded that "dose-dependent effects of violent head displacement in vulnerable brains predispose to dementia."[10]

Another review article makes a stronger argument for the relationship of TBI and Alzheimer's in moderate to severe TBI but

---

[10] M.F. Mendez, "What is the relationship of traumatic brain injury to dementia?" *Journal of Alzheimer's Disease*, 2017; 57(3): 667-681. doi: 10.3233/JAD-161002.

rightfully points out that there is little data for a link with mTBI, the most common type of concussion. It does make the point, however, that multiple but mild mTBIs, such as seen in boxers, football players, and hockey players, does lead to a specific type of dementia called chronic traumatic encephalopathy (CTE), as described in chapter 4. The article also states that the risk of developing Alzheimer's in moderate to severe TBI is increased two- to four-fold, but there is no data for mTBI.[11]

Yet another review expands the concept that trauma to the brain can cause different pathologies. The review makes an analogy between a single severe TBI and many cumulative mTBIs, both of which can contribute to developing CTE. The article also makes the point that TBI can contribute to several types of pathology, including different types of dementia and Parkinson's disease.[12]

In a 2015 study assessing the epidemiology of the association between mTBI and neurodegenerative disease, the authors describe a large study of 160,000 participants over the age of fifty-five. They found that patients who were aged sixty-five or older when they suffered a TBI had a 22 to 26 percent greater risk of developing dementia over the next five to seven years. However, the authors state that in younger subjects, who have greater healing capabilities, it could take longer than five to seven years for them to develop dementia.

The authors also reviewed the literature on the causation of Parkinson's disease from mTBI. They could find only five high-quality studies, three of which did not find any association. In the remaining two studies, the authors did find a positive association but questioned their own results; one study had poorly matched controls, and the other one attributed their results to "reverse causation." In a discussion of the epidemiology of CTE, they stress the point that the ability to develop Parkinson's disease from TBI is largely unknown

---

[11] S. Shively, et al., "Dementia resulting from traumatic brain injury: What is the pathology?" *Archives of Neurology*, 2012 Oct; 69(10): 1245-1251.

[12] P.M. Washington, et al., "Polypathology and dementia after brain trauma: Does brain injury trigger distinct neurodegenerative diseases, or should they be classified together as traumatic encephalopathy?" *Experimental Neurology*, 2016 Jan; 275 pt 3: 381-388. doi: 10.1016/j.expneurol.2015.06.015.

and cite numerous explanations for this (see table 2).

Table 2. Methodological Challenges of Epidemiological Studies of CTE.

Challenge	Consequence
Lack of consensus clinical criteria for CTE.	Prevalence/incidence can only be inferred from autopsy series, which are often limited by referral bias.
Variable definitions for mTBI used in prior studies.	Hinders comparison across studies.
Objective quantification/ measurement of repetitive mTBI exposure is difficult.	Population studied may have very heterogeneous mTBI exposures. Amount of mTBI exposure necessary to produce pathology is unknown.
Recall bias.	Symptomatic patients may be either more likely or less likely to recall mTBI exposure (if memory is affected).
Selection or referral bias.	Results are not broadly applicable to the general population.
Finding the appropriate control group is difficult.	Potential for confounding, as mTBI-exposed populations may differ from healthy controls in many ways besides mTBI exposure.
Secular trends: frequency and quality of mTBI exposure has changed dramatically among athletes and military personnel over the past century.	Unclear to what degree older studies may be applied to modern patients
Cohort effects: mTBI sustained in American football may differ considerably from mTBI sustained in boxing or combat.	Unclear to what degree studies of one cohort of patients exposed to repetitive mTBI may be applied to other cohorts.
CTE symptoms may not appear until years or decades following mTBI exposure.	Prospective studies from time of exposure to symptom onset may take decades to yield results. Retrospective studies may be influenced by recall bias or poorly quantified exposure.

Abbreviations: CTE = chronic traumatic encephalopathy; mTBI = mild traumatic brain injury

The authors also describe other risk factors for developing Parkinson's disease related to genetic factors, such as the genes coding for a protein that mutates and causes the association of Parkinson's disease after TBI. These genetic factors are made worse by certain pesticides (e.g., paraquat; see table 3).[13]

Table 3. Possible Risk Factors for Post-TBI Dementia, Parkinson's Disease, and CTE.

Risk Factor Category	Dementia	PD	CTE
Demographic	Increasing age	Increasing age	Increasing age
Genetic	APOE allele	Alpha-synuclein genotype	Competing results for APOE allele
TBI factors	More than one TBI	More than one TBI	Repetitive mTBI
	More severe TBI	More severe TBI	Repetitive sub-concussive head trauma
	Exposure to contact sports	Exposure to contact sports	Exposure and duration of exposure to contact sports
Other environmental exposures		Paraquat exposure	

Abbreviations: APOE = apolipoprotein; TBI = traumatic brain injury. Other abbreviations per table 2.

There are many more articles that I could cite, but the conclusions would be the same: there is probably enough data to say that a definite association between TBI and dementia has been established, with the recent discovery of CTE as an intermediary link. Since there is an association between CTE and dementia, the inference is more certain that the brain damage from concussions is an indirect cause of dementia.

[13] The last study and tables 2 and 3 are from R.C. Gardner and K. Yaffe, "Epidemiology of mild traumatic brain injury and neurodegenerative disease," *Molecular and Cellular Neuroscience*, 2015 May; 66 (Pt B): 75-80. doi: 10.1016/j.mcn.2015.03.001.

As for the concern for other potential neurodegenerative diseases, I do not believe that there is enough data to conclude a definite cause-and-effect relationship, although it may be just a question of time for the research to catch up and prove or disprove it. Personally, I do think it is possible that TBI can be related to the development of different neuro-degenerative diseases, but in my opinion, the treatment would be the same as described in Part II of this book. In any event, the best treatment for TBI is prevention.

For those who suffer a concussion (mTBI) and whose symptoms do not resolve (20 percent of patients), the best treatment is as I have described throughout the latter part of this book.

Chapter 15

Innovative New Treatments

There is not a lot of information available on innovative new treatments for TBI, but there is some. Distilling the information at hand, it appears to fall into two categories: 1) how to prevent concussions and 2) new forms of how to diagnose.

According to an article published in the Smithsonian magazine,[14] the University of Pennsylvania has developed a film that changes color on impact; the color corresponds to a specific amount of force. If someone were wearing a patch of the film on their head and was hit, for example, the film would record how much force the person's head had absorbed, which would then help to determine if enough force was applied to produce a concussion.

Anthony Gonzales, a former rugby player, has developed a mouthpiece called the FITGuard, which lights up when it is hit with enough force to cause a concussion. It can be ordered, but purchasers are placed on a waiting list. A company called X2 Biosystems has developed a patch that is placed behind the ear that also measures the force applied. Since up to 50 percent of sports players who sustain a concussion do not report it, this product should increase the opportunity to make more diagnoses of concussion. (The company was recently acquired by Prevent Biometrics.)

A professor at Harvard is studying the use of antibodies to help rid the brains of mice of misshapen tau proteins, the proteins that form as a result of experimentally induced concussion. He provides microscopic evidence that the treated mice's brains showed evidence of clearing the abnormal tau deposits. He states that his goal is for

---

[14] H. Hansman, "The Future of Concussions: How 5 New Advances Could Change Treatment," Smithsonian.com, 10 September 2015, last accessed 1 February 2019. See https://www.smithsonianmag.com/innovation/future-of-concussions-how-5-new-advances-could-change-treatment-180956543.

the technique to be adapted for humans.[15]

A novel method to assist in making the diagnosis of concussion is through using biomarkers, a measurable indicator to help determine the presence and severity of disease in the body. Biomarkers can come from the blood or spinal fluid, and from injury to the cell body or parts, glial support cells (cells in the central nervous system), and blood vessels.

Injury, especially the axonal type (DAI; discussed in chapter 1) in the brain's white matter, damages the axon and causes leakage of biomarker proteins, such as one called *neurofilament light*. These biomarkers correlate with the number of blows to the head in boxers.[16] The tau protein may be released from damage to unmyelinated fibers seen more in the grey matter, and it may be released in sub-concussive forces, too; pilot studies showed increases of plasma tau one hour after concussion in hockey players and persisting in military personnel who were deployed within the eighteen months prior to testing.

There are other biomarkers, many of which are of an esoteric nature, and the interested reader is referred to the article in the footnote on the Future Medicine website and other available literature. The conclusion to the biomarkers contribution is that the method is not fully developed enough at this time to be used in the clinical setting.

Functional MRI, known as fMRI, is a diagnostic tool that is used in a research setting to evaluate blood flow and oxygenation, known as the BOLD technique. It has been used to ascertain subtle changes in blood flow in sub-concussive-type injuries in high school football players. At this time, fMRI is available only at certain academic institutions performing that type of research and is not available to clinicians.

---

[15] M. Orcutt, "Will Football Players Someday Take a Concussion Pill?" *MIT Technology Review*, 22 July 2015, last accessed 1 February 2019. See https://www.technologyreview.com/s/539431/will-football-players-someday-take-a-concussion-pill.

[16] H. Zetterberg, et al., "Update on fluid biomarkers for concussion," *Concussion*, 2016; 1(3) CNC12. See https://www.futuremedicine.com/doi/pdf/10.2217/cnc-2015-0002.

Magnetoelectroencephalography, or MEG, measures the magnetic fields generated from the electric field produced by ordinary neuronal activity. Its main advantage is its time-based resolution, which is in milliseconds. Research has shown that MEG can detect delta waves in concussion that are also detected by QEEG. There are other variations of these techniques, and the interested reader is referred to scholarly articles on these methods.

At this point, I would like to add my own potential contribution in regard to improving and standardizing the treatment of TBI. The first step would be to perform a modern clinical trial (double-blind, placebo-controlled) of nimodipine for mTBI, since there are no published studies on this treatment. Based on my long and successful experience with this medication, the trial should be successful, and could therefore establish a new standard of treatment.

I have proposed an investigator-initiated clinical trial with the drug Nymalize, a brand name of nimodipine, to the drug manufacturer, Arbor Pharmaceuticals. I had a phone conference with the doctor in charge of clinical trials. He told me that the budget was fully allocated for the current year of 2019 but that if I could secure financing, then Arbor Pharmaceuticals would be willing to donate the medication for the trial. He also said that he may be interested in performing a clinical trial for 2020 but that he would have to confer with his team. As of 06-19, I have not heard from Arbor Pharmaceuticals.

Another potential clinical trial is to evaluate the difference of efficacy of nimodipine alone vs. nimodipine with magnesium, the latter of which would ensure that proper red blood cell magnesium levels are maintained. Yet another theoretical study is to modify the structure of nimodipine to see if it could be made more effective than the parent molecule.

I recently came across an exciting potential new treatment. It is in the laboratory stage of testing now but holds great promise. Researchers added relatively simple molecules to human glial support cells in cell cultures. They injected the modified human cells into mice, which then lived for another month. These chemicals induced the glial cells to transform into neurons, including establishing new synaptic connections.[17] The implications for recovery are enormous.

I think that the future treatment for TBI looks fairly good. Advances are being made on many fronts, but the traditional treatment aspect is clearly lacking. My protocol, on the other hand, has made significant strides forward. Getting my message out to the medical community and the public at large will make the future of treatment look even brighter.

---

[17] B. Kennedy, "Chemical transformation of glial cells into neurons," medical research, Pennsylvania State University, 15 October 2015.

Chapter 16

Hope for Past, Current, and Future Patients with TBI

Throughout this book I have endeavored to convey the message that there is a comprehensive treatment available that can reverse all the symptoms of a concussion, even though it is not well known or established in the literature.

With this book, it is my greatest hope that more people with TBI will know about and have access to treatment that can and does repair injuries to the brain, regardless of whether the injury is current or happened long ago. As documented in the four case studies in chapter 13, I have seen thousands of dramatic recoveries with my patients, and there is every reason to believe that if you apply the same methods of treatment, then you or your loved one can also recover from concussion.

The critical point is that once the two basic diagnostic tests are obtained, the treatment that follows will allow your brain to heal. All patients should strive to empower themselves, and you now have the formula to make that happen. While some physicians may not be familiar with the information I have shared with you, there is much medical and scientific information to share with them if they are not comfortable ordering the tests or writing a prescription for an FDA-approved medication. Samples of how QEEG and SPECT scan prescriptions should be written are provided in chapter 7. Give a copy of them to your personal physician. I am always available to chat or correspond with your treating physician, should the occasion arise.

My website has much information on concussion and treatment, including a blog and a podcast. One purpose for the latter two is to provide the most up-to-date methods of treating and reversing symptoms from a concussion, as discussed throughout this book. In fact, I have recently learned of a new anti-aging technique that may be applied to treating concussions with a different approach. I am confident that there will be many more new discoveries as time passes, and I shall always be on the lookout for new and innovative ways to treat and heal a concussion.

I believe that the future of concussion and TBI treatment is very bright, and that all past, present, and prospective patients can have a high probability of meaningful recovery.

CONCUSSIONS CAN BE HEALED

The brain is a remarkable organ, unique in its functions and capabilities. New neurons can grow and new synapses form, thus literally growing new brain matter. Those who are wheelchair-bound from a head injury may be able to walk again. Poor cognitive function can be repaired. Muscle strength and reflexes can return. In fact, all symptoms can be improved if not totally reversed.

The diagnostic tools discussed in this book, SPECT, QEEG, and QEP, reveal previously hidden brain injuries that can go undetected for years, even decades. Subtle cognitive dysfunction may be a direct result of such an injury, and until now, most people have had to just live with it. Many people never discover that their loss of cognitive function is a from a head trauma. Correct diagnosis is key to unmasking the injury so that it can be treated and healed.

Unfortunately, most physicians are not aware of the treatments for mTBI and TBI that are discussed in this book. It is vitally important that patients are actively engaged in their own treatment, and you are now better informed to have discussions with your physician on the diagnosis and treatment of concussion. Be firm, ask for what you want, and don't stop until you get it. Your brain's health depends on it.

The treatments I have described throughout this book have been proven over and over by the thousands of patients I have treated. Nimodipine works to bring blood flow back to normal, or close to it, in the brain's injured tissues. Neurofeedback works by virtue of the brain's neuroplasticity, its ability to correct abnormal brain waves. It is not a difficult treatment, and patients may even enjoy it. Hyperbaric oxygen therapy delivers oxygen-rich air to the body through the lungs, tissues, and many other mechanisms. The oxygen-rich blood, supported by the increased blood flow from the nimodipine, floods the brain, allowing it to help heal the injuries.

There is hope for every person suffering the effects of concussion. The brain can be healed. It takes determination, dedication, and working with a physician who supports you in your quest for optimal health. Never give up in your quest to heal your brain.

Appendix A

Why QEEG Is Underutilized by Neurologists

As demonstrated throughout chapter 7, it is clear that QEEG is a superior diagnostic test compared to the standard EEG, which is read by visual interpretation. So why then is QEEG not in the mainstream of diagnostic tests by neurologists and other physicians who order EEGS? The answer is certainly not based on scientifically valid reasons, but rather on politics, failure to teach the test procedure in medical schools, and position statements by official groups such as the American Academy of Neurology.

In general, medical doctors become members of various local and national associations like the American Medical Association, commonly called the AMA. Most specialities have their own speciality organization on state and nationwide bases. Neurologists even have two national associations that they may belong to. The one that I was introduced to as a young resident is the American Academy of Neurology, or AAN, and I was a member for many years.

Most national groups, including the AAN, publish a monthly journal that most physicians read as much as possible to keep up with new research, since private practitioners like me are no longer affiliated with university centers, where all new information stems from. The AAN publishes a monthly magazine with peer-reviewed articles that include new research and clinical trials of drugs or devices to either diagnose or treat various neurological conditions. Most neurologists take these publications very seriously and consider the information as valid. They depend on the veracity and accuracy of what is promulgated.

The AAN produces what they call *position statements* to inform the general population of neurologists what its opinion is on any given subject. These position statements are taken most seriously by practitioners, since they are written by academicians who are in a more powerful position by virtue of their academic appointment. Thus, the statements issued by the AAN are considered to be gospel by practicing neurologists like me, who have to see patients every day to earn a living. We often say that the academicians live and work in an ivory tower because of the unique position they are in and the enormous impact their opinions and thus position statements have on local practitioners like me, who are sometimes described as working in the trenches.

It is appropriate to review the position statements by AAN, which have been authored by Mark Nuwer, MD, PhD, a professor of neurology at UCLA since the 1970s. He is also the director of the clinical neurophysiology program at the university. Neurophysiology refers to the functioning of the nervous system, and covers many different types of diagnostic testing, from the brain down to the feet.

Starting in 1989, the first of several position statements were published and authored by Dr. Nuwer. The following conclusion is copied here for a starting point in the debate, which ensued after its publication in August of that year: "Executive summary. EEG brain mapping is of limited usefulness in clinical neurology. The tests are best used by physicians highly skilled in EEG, in conjunction with analysis of the concurrent polygraph EEG." I interpreted this statement as a neutral one, and that as long as a trained neurologist followed the rules, it was all right to use the test for any type of patient.

Another prestigious national organization called at the time the American Electroencephalography Association (AMEEGA) disagreed with the AAN's position and published their official announcement in their journal, *Clinical Electroencephalography*, in 1996 (vol. 27, no. 2). The members and editorial staff of this journal are epileptologists, that is, neurologists with additional expertise in EEG/QEEG and in treating epilepsy. Their statement was highly critical of the 1989 statement by Nuwer for a number of reasons, but especially because of errors, especially that of omission.

Among this type of error was cited the lack of mention of scientific papers on QEEG that had been published over the previous thirty years. They also pointed out a frank error of omission in that the 1989 paper used the terms *QEEG* and *brain mapping* synonymously, but the words are not synonymous. They go on to point out that after the 1980s, when brain mapping was popularized by the manufactures of the instruments, the statement was irresponsible because it contributed to damaging the good name of QEEG. Their favorable view on QEEG was in accordance with the National Advisory Mental Health Council (NAMHC), the nation's highest-level independent board, which published a statement and reported to the United States Congress.

NAMHC's conclusion was that the QEEG was recommended in six different clinical categories, and even stated that in the fourth category of "organic mental syndromes," the QEEG "must be applied in every patient diagnosed with this syndrome." Many conditions were included in this subcategory, including one called *post-traumatic organic brain syndrome*. In other diagnostic terms, the latter condition would be synonymous with concussion/post-concussion syndrome.

My personal interpretation of the AMEEGA position statement was that I agreed with it wholeheartedly, and I felt vindicated using the test. Over the years, I have defended many plaintiffs through depositions. I was often asked about the AAN position statement, and I responded with the AMEEGA statement. I also testified that between the two divergent opinions, I chose the AMEEGA's position, citing that epileptologists were more knowledgeable on matters of EEG/QEEG, and I deferred to their judgment and not that of the AAN.

Several explanations were offered for the position of the AAN (even though the AAN did not offer any themselves). These included bias by omitting a psychiatrist on the committee that published the statement, and bias of excluding relevant articles in the scientific literature, especially those concerning the use of QEEG by pharmaceutical companies, who were conducting the procedure for many years prior to the advent of brain mapping to determine the precise effects of medications on the brain's electrical patterns. There were many other comments along similar lines of thought, which are not included here since they are beyond the scope of this discussion.

In July 1997, *Neurology*, the official journal of the AAN, also known as the "Green Journal," Dr. Nuwer published a second position statement. This newer statement was much more detailed, as he described some of the benefits and advantages of QEEG over EEG and listed a number of neurological conditions for which QEEG would be an appropriate test—and when it may not be appropriate. Once again, he did not offer an explanation for the conditions that were excluded.

He also listed a number of conditions for which "QEEG remains investigational for clinical use [including] post-concussion syndrome, mild or moderate head injury, learning disability, attention disorders," and other conditions. He went to write, "On the basis of clinical and scientific evidence, opinions of most experts, and the technical and methodologic shortcomings, QEEG is not recommended for use in civil or criminal judicial proceedings." He concluded, "Because of the very substantial risk of erroneous interpretations, it is unacceptable for any EEG brain mapping or other QEEG techniques to be used clinically by those who are not physicians highly skilled in clinical EEG interpretation." Unfortunately, again, he never cited a reason or rationale for excluding the relevant topic of TBI.

At the time of this position statement, I had been performing QEEG for about twelve years and had studied several thousand patients, most of whom had sustained head trauma with concussion. My opinion was that the tests were highly appropriate and useful in evaluating patients, especially when the routine tests were normal. I could never understand how an expert in EEG and QEEG and the director of an entire neurophysiology department could offer an opinion that was so contrary to my training and hands-on experience.

Outraged by this second statement, several authors contributed to an article that appeared one month later in the *Journal of Neuropsychiatry and Clinical Neurosciences* titled "Limitations of the American Academy of Neurology and American Clinical Neurophysiology Society paper on QEEG." Of the authors, one name in particular stood out: that of Robert Thatcher, PhD, who is the creator of the *NeuroGuide*, a software program used to create QEEG data files on my patients, including the ones reproduced with permission in this book. Dr. Thatcher also helped create and write software to perform neurofeedback, the therapy discussed in chapter 9. The introductory paragraph to the article is powerful and informative:

A committee of experts, including physicians and psychologists, has drafted this response to the American Academy of Neurology and American Clinical Neurophysiology Society's (AAN/ACNS) paper "Assessment of Digital EEG, Quantitative EEG, and EEG Brain Mapping," edited by Dr. Marc Nuwer. It is the opinion of this committee, supported by the leadership of the Association for Applied Psychophysiology and Biofeedback (AAPB) and the Society for the Study of Neuronal Regulation (SSNR), that the AAN/ACNS report is biased and contains factual errors. This committee, as a body representing AAPB and SSNR, is concerned about the accuracy of the report, its scope, and the damage that it may cause in the health care and science fields. The AAN/ACNS conclusions, as they are currently written, should not be considered the definitive opinion on digital EEG.[18]

The report goes on to criticize the 1997 report in that "the basis on which the 'positively recommended' group was selected in comparison to the 'negatively recommended' group is not evident in the AAN/ACNS report, and this dichotomous classification

[18] DA Hoffman, et al., "Limitations of the American Academy of Neurology and American Clinical Neurophysiology Society paper on QEEG," *Journal of Neuropsychiatry and Clinical Neurosciences*, 1999 Summer; 11(3): 401-407.

lacks a serious scientific foundation. For example, the criterion of prospective verification was not equally applied to the 'accepted' QEEG applications and the 'rejected' applications. Indeed, the report appears incomplete in that it misrepresents the literature and omits citations that support scientific opposing views concerning the 'clinically rejected' categories."

The article goes on to describe different biases and points out factual errors that led to erroneous conclusions. They pointed out how the 1997 paper was misleading and how Nuwer contradicted his own conclusions. They stated that the paper was not scientifically balanced and that the true accuracy and utility of QEEG was not properly recognized. If it were not a valid test, why would four VA hospitals and three military bases employ QEEG on a regular basis to veterans returning with TBI?

The authors conclude their paper with this summary: "The AAN/ACNS report is misleadingly negative regarding the current status of quantitative EEG and tends to discourage its development and use with other related clinical problems. There have been many excellent studies showing that QEEG can be useful for the evaluation and understanding of mild traumatic brain injury, learning disabilities, attention deficit disorders, alcoholism, depression, and other types of substance abuse. In fact, Hughes and John recently provided in this Journal an extensive and detailed review of the use of QEEG in psychiatric disorders."

While the saga of the official story as to why QEEG is not considered to be the routine test to order is over and done with, there is an unofficial story that has an unsavory ending worthy of mention. In medico-legal cases, as we all know, there are two sides involved with the proceedings, namely the plaintiff, who is the injured party, and the defendant, who is charged with harming the plaintiff. Each party is typically represented by legal counsel. The resolution of the case is either settled out of court or must be fought in court. I am quite familiar with the process, since I have testified as an expert witness many times since 1985, typically for the plaintiff side.

This unsavory story commences with a personal injury case in the state of New York. The plaintiff was diagnosed with a concussion, and the treating physician assessed the TBI with a QEEG. The defense made a motion to disallow the QEEG data, citing that it was not an accepted test and should be stricken from the record. The defense provided an expert witness to confirm that the QEEG should not be used in cases of trauma because it was not recommended by the AAN.

It was no coincidence that the expert witness produced by the defense was none other than Mark Nuwer, the author of the highly criticized position statement. The plaintiff's attorney discovered that the QEEG data that Dr. Nuwer provided during testimony under oath was in fact quantified data from artifactual data (such as from an eye blink) but that Nuwer failed to tell the judge, thus misleading the judge and jury into believing that the QEEG data was not valid.

He also showed that if the data was processed on several occasions (he showed four examples), the results were not identical as (he said) they should be, but that is not physiologically possible. He had, in fact, pre-prepared samples of four different artifacts from an unsuspecting doctor who thought the data was being used to teach how *not* to perform QEEG. Needless to say, such conduct and behavior are completely unacceptable and certainly far below any standard of medical care.

As a result of Dr. Nuwer's unethical behavior, a formal complaint was filed against him claiming "1: Intentional misrepresentation to a State Supreme Court Judge about facts concerning medical diagnostic technology with implication for patient's right for proper evaluation and care. 2: Misrepresentation of educational degrees and methods in regard to Mr. Gunkelman. [Gunkelman, an accomplice in the case, misled a doctor into thinking that an FFT artifact was for teaching purposes and not for official testimony in the trial.] 3: False or misleading statements or omissions of a material nature. 4: Interference with a patient's right for due process, compensation in a court of law."

Clearly, not many physicians, including doctorate-level therapists, know the value of QEEG in diagnosing TBI. This is a problem that needs to be corrected but will take considerable effort. A step in that direction is to convince medical schools to begin teaching QEEG and the concept that QEEG is one of many tests used to evaluate brain electrical function. Another possibility is to establish teaching seminars, webinars, and other educational formats that include continuing medical education credits for physicians already in practice. Similar comments can be made about the use of SPECT scans to diagnose TBI and the use of HBOT in the treatment of TBI.

Appendix B

Why HBOT Is Underutilized

As you will learn in this section, the use of HBOT for TBI and other injuries is not as common as it could be, considering its benefits.

Most of the following information comes from an article entitled "All the right moves: the need for the timely use of hyperbaric oxygen therapy for treating TBI/CTE/PTSD" (*Medical Gas Research*, 2015; 5:7) by Dr. Kenneth P. Stoller, the chief of Hyperbaric Medicine, Hyperbaric Oxygen Clinic of San Francisco.

Dr. Stoller writes that even though HBOT has been around since 1937, it is not well known. He contrasts this against the sobering fact that every day, an average of twenty US military veterans commit suicide related to TBI and post-traumatic stress disorder (PTSD), the two signature injuries from the wars in Iraq and Afganistan.

He writes that there is no question that HBOT is effective in treating TBI/PTSD, but it is being denied to veterans. He writes, "Every suicide might be seen as a tremendous cost saving to certain technocrats." He describes an "unspoken rationale" that if the military were to advocate that veterans should be treated with HBOT for their injuries, then current active troops would come forward to get their treatment, leading to troop strength being decimated because so many would be in treatment.

He further states that in order to delay the acceptance of HBOT as a valid form of treatment, the Department of Defense (DOD) has deliberately funded false studies. The DOD has also claimed that low-pressure air is the same as a placebo (it is not), and that there is no difference when comparing a placebo with treatment (there is). The civilian trials of HBOT for TBI are all favorable, as was one

Israeli military study, whereas all of the DOD-sponsored studies do not show any benefit. Clearly, one side of these divergent opinions is right, and the other is just wrong. You can draw your own conclusion.

Dr. Stoller points out that HBOT is considered the "Cinderella of conventional medicine" because, despite the fact that it has been proven as an effective treatment for many conditions, HBOT is "treated with derision or ignored at best." Pharmaceutical companies will not pay for expensive clinical trials because HBOT is not patentable, and thus there is no pot of gold to be made, as there is with blockbuster drugs.

His argument is raised to a higher and more ethical level when he points out that the twenty veterans a day who commit suicide related to TBI/PTSD exceeds the losses in active combat. The issue of suicide also includes the former NFL players described in chapter 4.

Fortunately, a clinical trial called the National Brain Injury Rescue & Rehabilitation project (NBIRR) showed that HBOT "can virtually eliminate suicidality in this population once they are treated with HBOT, while reducing depression by 51%."[19]

Dr. Stollar criticizes the use of antidepressants (SSRIs) to treat TBI/PTSD for various reasons, such as side effects and the lack of efficacy. They cause neuronal damage and trigger mature neurons to revert to an immature state, both of which may contribute to cell apoptosis. He notes that HBOT has prevented death in acute severe TBI by 59 percent, a huge accomplishment the likes of which has not been seen since the discovery of penicillin, the invention of the ambulance, and the use of helicopters in Vietnam to treat battle injuries (like MASH in Korea). The big question, then, is, why hasn't HBOT become the standard of care? What could be the reasons behind this enigma?

Part of the problem has to do with financial matters. As already mentioned, pharmaceutical companies will not play a role in the

---

[19] Vance H. Trimble, *The Uncertain Miracle: Hyperbaric Oxygen, the Little-Known Maverick Medical Treatment which Has Saved the Lives of Thousands of People*. Doubleday, 1974.

development of HBOT because there is no money for them to make.

The NBIRR project, which treats returning veterans with HBOT, has seen an outstanding success rate of 60 to 80 percent of treated vets who are able to return to work or school. Dr. Stoller further asserts that for every veteran who is treated with HBOT and returns to active duty, the government saves $2.6 million, and for each soldier who returns to civilian work or school, the government saves $2 million. He then asks why the government won't treat all veterans with HBOT. His proposes that a sinister reason lies beneath the surface: showing that HBOT is not an effective treatment may be a cover-up for the fact that if a veteran does commit suicide, then the cost to the government is zero dollars.

Dr. Stoller makes a compelling case that what the DOD is doing (or not doing) to veterans is analagous to what the NFL has done to their former and current players: withhold the truth that concussions cause brain damage and lead to chronic traumatic encephalopathy (CTE), which results in behavioral and cognitive issues, all of which may contribute to suicide.

The fact that the NFL intentionally and fraudulently hid the truth of the medical facts has led to a class-action lawsuit against the organization and continues to be widely publicized. Big corporations continue to deny and obscure the truth, and this seems to be the way this country is moving forward, to the detriment of the public. As examples, we can look at the history of the tobacco industry denying and obscuring the dangers of smoking cigarettes and corporate denial of asbestos causing mesothelioma. Both of these instances required class-action litigation to resolve, resulting in multi-billion dollar settlements. To this day, lawyers advertise on TV that if your loved one was exposed to asbestos, you can still file a lawsuit and collect compensation, even if that person has passed on.

The NFL continues to deny benefits to its former players through a program called the 88 Plan, which is intended to assist vested former players with dementia. Recall that concussions are cumulatively damaging to the brain, especially when players are sent back to play and then receive another concussion before recovering from the first one. This is called second-impact syndrome, and it contributes to dementia with or without CTE. Since the position of the NFL is that CTE does not cause dementia, if a player is diagnosed with CTE, they are not eligible for benefits, and thus they are denied coverage to receive HBOT. Once again, the tactics of denial and hiding the truth seem to be the determining factors in deciding and making important policies, to the detriment of the players who need it most, just as with veterans.

Dr. Stoller summarizes his article by stating why HBOT is not adopted: because it cannot be patented and does not have a large corporate sponsor despite being an effective, benign, and humanitarian approach to treating TBI/PTSD. He reiterates the interference of accepting HBOT as the standard of care by "maintaining the status quo, myopic budgetary constraints, or perceived liability issues." Lastly, he points out that the general public is being misled and that the average person does not know that medical decisions are made by technocrats instead of professionals with the medical knowledge and wisdom to choose what is best for veterans and anyone suffering from TBI/PTSD.

I will add my own opinion and say for the record that the travesty and lack of appropriate treatment of all of our soldiers, whether active or inactive, and in fact anyone suffering from TBI/PTSD, needs to be exposed on a large-scale level—including by conducting official congressional hearings—and once and for all letting the truth be told. Too many individuals have suffered too many conditions because the responsible parties do not want to pay up.

It is the patient's right to be afforded the best possible treatment. If you, the empowered patient, want to get HBOT, you can do so by asking for a prescription from any licensed doctor who is willing to write it. If your doctor refuses, then all HBOT centers have a supervisory physician whom you can see, and that doctor will be happy to write or just authorize the treatment. All HBOT centers treat all types of wounds, including wounds to the brain, such as a TBI.

Glossary

amplitude: The size of a response, usually measured in microvolts.

angiogenesis: The creation of new blood vessels (arteries, arterioles).

anterior: Toward the front.

aphasia: A disorder of language, either impaired speaking or impaired understanding, or both.

apoptosis: The death of a cell.

arterioles: Small-caliber arteries.

atrophy: Shrinkage, loss of cells.

axon: A single fiber carrying information from the cell body.

biofeedback: A process by which a person can retrain a bodily function.

biomarker: A diagnostic test to determine a specific bodily function.

blood-brain barrier (BBB): A protective barrier around cerebral vessels to prevent toxins from entering the brain.

brainstem: A relay structure carrying information from the brain to the body and from the body to the brain.

cerebral cortex: The most advanced part of the brain; it is the largest in humans and is what makes humans intelligent.

chronic traumatic encephalopathy (CTE): Physical damage to the brain following concussion.

commissures: Connections of white matter from left to right or from front to back in the brain.

coup contrecoup injury: A trauma pattern in the brain seen in damaged areas after concussion, for example, left front and right back areas.

diffuse axonal injury (DAI): A pattern of injury, a twisting of the brain, damaging the junction of the grey and the white matter.

dura mater: A dense, fibrous tissue close to the skull; one of the protective linings of the brain.

edema: Swelling of the brain from various sources, including trauma.

EEG: Electroencephalography; a diagnostic test to measure the brain waves, in which sensors are attached to the scalp.

epidemiology: The scientific study of the occurrence of natural occurrences.

epidural hematoma: A dangerous blood clot outside the brain that needs surgery to remove in order to save the victim's life.

focal: One part of the brain.

focal seizure: A seizure starting from one part of the brain.

grey matter: The outer surface of the brain containing neurons and their connections; it is most highly developed in humans.

hemorrhagic DAI: A diffuse axonal injury with bleeding at the junction of the grey matter and the white matter.

herniation: A compression of one part of the brain, pushing it down into the bottom of the brain, causing coma and death if not reversed.

hypoperfusion: Decreased blood flow in the brain or other organs.

infarction: Dead tissue from loss of oxygen; comes from blockage of an artery or spasm of same.

inner table: The inside surface of the skull.

ischemia: The lack of oxygen as a result of decreased blood flow.

latency: The time from the onset of a stimulus to the recorded response of the brain or other nervous tissue, usually measured in milliseconds.

lateralization: Refers to one side, or hemisphere, of the brain.

liposoluble: A substance that readily dissolves in fat or mostly fatty substance.

lobes of the brain –

frontal lobe: The front of the brain; largest in humans and performs executive function, intelligence, and the ability to speak verbally.

occipital lobe: At the back of the brain, responsible for vision.

parietal lobe: At the middle of the brain, responsible for math functions, sequencing, left-right orientation, and spatial representation.

temporal lobe: At the bottom middle of the brain, responsible for language and memory.

LORETA: An EEG extension enabling analysis of the function of deep electrical activity of the brain.

mild traumatic brain injury (mTBI): Physical trauma to the brain; concussion, usually with no loss of consciousness.

morbidity: Any medical condition that causes disease; also called co-morbidity or multiple conditions.

motor aphasia: Impairment of the ability to speak.

neocortex: A part of the cortex, most highly developed in humans; has six layers of cells.

neurofeedback: A method of treating the brain to correct underlying abnormal brain waves.

neuronal dysfunction: Any condition wherein a nerve cell does not work properly.

neuroplasticity: The ability of the brain waves to change; used in neurofeedback to repair brain waves.

non-hemorrhagic DAI: Damage at the grey-white matter without bleeding.

normative database: A collective of data from a group without pathology or abnormal conditions.

perfusion: Blood flow.

peripheral edema: Swelling of the extremities.

post-concussion syndrome: A myriad of symptoms after sustaining a concussion.

posterior: Toward the back or the back of an organ or body part.

QEEG: Quantitative electroencephalography; computerized EEG.

QEP: Quantitative evoked potentials; stimulation and recording of different sensory systems, such as visual, auditory, and cognitive.

secondary injury: A second injury that occurs before the first injury is healed.

SPECT scan: A type of scan that shows blood flow in various organs.

subarachnoid hemorrhage: A type of bleeding in the brain in the subarachnoid space.

traumatic brain injury (TBI): An injury to the brain from direct or indirect acceleration/deceleration applied to the brain, with or without loss of consciousness.

white matter: The part of the brain that conveys, sends, and receives messages.

Made in the USA
Columbia, SC
21 January 2020

86969750R00109